Extraordinary Healing Secrets

from a

Doctor's Private Files

JAMES K. VAN FLEET, D.C.

Parker Publishing Company, Inc.

West Nyack, New York

©1977, *by*

James K. Van Fleet, D.C.

Library of Congress Cataloging in Publication Data

Van Fleet, James K
    Extraordinary healing secrets from a doctor's private files.

    Includes index.
    1. Diet in disease.   2. Vitamin therapy.   I. Title.
RM217.V29   615'.854   76-28517
ISBN 0-13-298190-4

Printed in the United States of America

Dedication

*This book is dedicated to three people
I love very much...*

my daughter's husband,

G. Arch Spain

and my two grandsons,

Adam Lucas Spain
Joel Van Spain

Also by the author ...

Doctor Van Fleet's Amazing New "Non-Glue-Food" Diet,
James K. Van Fleet, D.C., 1974, Parker.

What This Book Will Do for You

If you are one of the millions of Americans who use anti-acids for your heartburn and upset stomach...laxatives for your constipation...aspirin for your headache...pain killers for your arthritis and rheumatism...pep pills to stay awake and feel energetic...sleeping pills for your insomnia...tranquilizers for your nervous tension...and suppositories for your hemorrhoids, then this book is for you. It will show you how to get over these conditions so you won't need to take those drugs anymore.

I'm sure you know by now that these various medicines and drugs do not cure disease. They treat only the symptoms to give you a temporary fleeting relief without any lasting benefits whatever. If you've become discouraged with that kind of treatment in a futile attempt to gain back your good health and get well again, then I repeat: *this book is for you.*

Or if you've been troubled with some chronic condition that seems to defy orthodox medical treatment or drug medication, it could well be that you'll find the answer to your specific problem right here in these pages. For instance, Chapters 1 through 4 cover a wide variety of ailments that have been helped by my extraordinary methods of using natural foods, vitamins, minerals, enzymes and herbs.

Chapter 5 deals specifically with how you can get rid of colds, hay fever, allergies, sinus problems and other respiratory ailments. Chapters 6 and 7 cover upper and lower digestive tract problems and show you how to take care of canker sores, bleeding gums, gas pains, gastritis and heartburn, constipation, diarrhea, ulcerative colitis, diverticulitis, rectal itching, and hemorrhoids.

Chapter 8 shows you that you don't have to suffer with the aches and pains of arthritis and rheumatism, while Chapter 9 discusses how to get rid of headaches, insomnia and nervous tension with new and remarkable healing methods. Chapter 10 reveals how you can deal with various skin conditions so you can have a glowing, youthful and radiant complexion.

Chapter 11 discusses the secrets of how to keep your heart and circulation young and vital, and Chapter 12 explores all the details of that mysterious and frustrating malady — hypoglycemia or low blood sugar — and shows you how to correct or prevent that condition with safe, easy, and quick drugless methods. Chapter 13 tells you how to avoid or correct the special problems of older age easily, safely and painlessly, while the last chapter gives you the outstanding methods my own patients use to keep from getting sick again once they're well.

As you read, you'll be able to see for yourself how my extraordinary methods are effective in correcting long standing cases of asthma, sinusitis, arthritis, rheumatism, low back pain, indigestion, heartburn, constipation, diarrhea, circulatory conditions, insomnia, headache, nervous exhaustion and many, many others.

You'll be able to read one thrilling case history after another taken right from my private files that show the efficacy of my methods in combatting chronic illness. For instance, you'll meet Nancy, whose nervous tension was cleared up in two short weeks...Frank, who got rid of his hemorrhoids without painful surgery...Margaret, whose miserable migraine headaches were quickly relieved after 25 years of torture...Marlene, whose early glaucoma was miraculously reversed...Jerry, who got rid of his nagging backache as if by magic...Tom, a pharmacist, who cured his sore throat by using my natural methods... George, whose heartburn and gastritis were cured in only one week after a year and a half of suffering...Sarah, who got complete relief from ten long years of constipation...Lucy, who recovered completely even though her entire life was threatened by rheumatoid arthritis and many, many more.

These people, all patients of mine, gained these remark-able results not with drugs and surgery, but by following the extraordinary guidelines to good health that are given in this book. It is my sincere desire that you will be able to enjoy similar benefits for yourself. If you follow the recommendations and suggestions I've set forth here, I feel confident that you will.

* * *

Before beginning Chapter 1, I would like to cover a few important details here that will help you in your understanding and total enjoyment of my book.

First of all, the vitamins, minerals and food supplements I discuss are to be taken in either *capsule* or *tablet* form. Unless I specifically say that the item is to be taken as a liquid or pow-der, you will know it is always a tablet or capsule.

For instance, if I say you should take 2,000 grams of calcium a day, the number of tablets you would take would depend on the amount of calcium in each one. I usually recom-mend that calcium be taken in the form of *dolomite*. Now some manufacturers put 130 milligrams in each tablet; others put 158; still others, 214. No two companies are ever quite alike. So you must first of all read the label to see the amount of calcium contained in each tablet of dolomite before you know how many tablets you need to take a day.

Dolomite also contains magnesium, but you need pay no attention whatever to the amount. You see, dolomite contains calcium and magnesium in their natural ratio, approximately two to one. So when you take the amount of calcium you need, you will automatically get the proper amount of magnesium with it.

Vitamin C is another example. Let's suppose I recommend 3,000 milligrams of vitamin C each day. It can be purchased in all kinds of assorted sizes: 100, 250, 300, 500, or even 1,000 milligram tablets. Which of these you use does not matter at all as long as the total amount is correct. For instance, sometimes you'll find that one particular size is on sale. Naturally, that would be the one to buy. Usually, the larger the milligram size of the tablet the more economical the vitamin is. A 1,000 milli-gram tablet of vitamin C is much less expensive than four 250 milligram tablets. However, if you were only taking 1,000 milligrams of vitamin C a day, you would be better off to take a 250 milligram tablet four times a day rather than a 1,000 milligram tablet only once since the body gets more value and assimilates more of the food supplement when it is taken several times a day.

So I usually recommend to my patients that they take their food supplements three or four times a day. Now if I ask you to take a particular vitamin, mineral, or food supplement three times a day, that means you should take it at breakfast, dinner and supper. If I were to say to take it four times a day, then the fourth time would be bed time.

Vitamins and minerals should normally not be taken on an empty stomach. They should be consumed when you have just eaten or a few at a time during the course of your meal. Any liquid, fruit juice, water or milk — your preference — is quite satisfactory to wash them down.

Vitamins A, D, and E are oil soluble and usually come in the form of a gelatine capsule. Vitamins B and C are water soluble and normally come in a tablet form. But as usual, there are always those exceptions. For instance, in my office shelf supply, I have some vitamin A tablets and some vitamin B capsules. The important thing to keep in mind is the total amount you're getting. As a matter of interest and clarification, the oil soluble vitamins — A, D, and E — are always measured in *units*. The water soluble ones — the B complex and C — are always measured in *milligrams*.

All your vitamins should be *natural* or *organic* rather than synthetic. You see, nutrients in nature do not occur alone. For instance, if you were to take the synthetic vitamin C, you would get only *ascorbic acid*. But in vitamin C made from organic sources, you would get not only ascorbic acid but also all other trace elements, enzyme catalysts, and other nutritional substances that compose the totality of vitamin C as found in nature.

To get the entire B complex — which contains at least 11 vitamins that are widely accepted (others no doubt exist that have not yet been discovered or isolated) — you must take the natural vitamin. Organic vitamins condensed from natural foods contain many interrelated nutrients. They are considered to be much safer and better for maintaining your good health than synthetics.

Therefore, I would strongly recommend that you purchase all your vitamins and minerals such as *zinc, dolomite, iron, sea kelp,* etc. in a reliable health food store that you trust, or by mail order from one of the vitamin and mineral companies that advertise in *Prevention,* the monthly health magazine published by the Rodale Press, Inc., Emmaus, Pennsylvania, 18049.

Vitamins and minerals can be purchased from any of these companies with complete confidence. There are too many government agencies — the Federal Trade Commission, Interstate Commerce Commission, Postmaster General, Federal Food and Drug Administration — monitoring and checking their activities for them to be unreliable.

Prevention magazine also is extremely careful about the advertising it accepts. Vitamin companies who use synthetics to make their products cannot advertise in *Prevention.* Besides requiring adequate laboratory test reports from their advertisers, *Prevention* is constantly spot-checking products through independent laboratory analyses. Their guidelines are frequently higher than government standards for comparable products, and their enforcement procedures result in the rejection of many pages of advertising each year.

I myself use the vitamin and mineral products from many of the companies who advertise in *Prevention.* You should compare prices of their products so you can save money. Many of them run specials and that's the best time to buy. Vitamins and minerals by mail order are usually less expensive than the exact same products in your health food store, for you're getting them directly from the manufacturer.

I do not recommend one company above another, but I must say that *Puritan's Pride* is the only natural vitamin and mineral company I've found to date who manufacturers the vitamin B complex from *organic sources* in the high potencies I recommend for my patients. For instance, their *B-50,* which is a balanced super potency of B complex vitamins in the 50 milligram range, supplies ten to fifteen times the potency of the average natural B complex vitamin formula. Their *B-100* has twice as much as their *B-50*.

They also make the individual vitamins of the B complex in high potencies — 100 milligrams and above — so my patients can increase their intake of Thiamin, Riboflavin, Niacin, Pyridoxine, Choline, Inositol, Pantothenic Acid and so on, based on their own individual needs.

Their address is 105 Orville Drive, Bohemia, New York, 11716. If you write them, I'm sure they'll be glad to send you a copy of their current catalog. Before doing so, check their address in a current issue of *Prevention* in case it might have been changed.

Other companies, usually manufacturers of drugs and pharmaceuticals, do make the vitamin B complex in high potencies, but their products are usually available only to the doctor or the retail pharmacy where they are often sold by prescription only. Not only that, they are *not* natural vitamins from organic sources, but *synthetics*.

So then. With these important points in mind now, let's get right on to Chapter 1 and the first exciting case history.

James K. Van Fleet, D.C.

Contents

How I cleared up Nancy's nervous problems in two short
weeks with this amazing new treatment • How Sam, my
mailman, got rid of his blistered feet with my unusually
easy-to-use treatment • Why my treatment is considered
to be unorthodox and unconventional • How Anna quickly
got rid of her canker sores with my unique procedures
• How Frank amazingly eliminated his hemmorhoids
without painful surgery in only 48 hours • Margaret's
migraine headaches incredibly relieved after 25 years of
misery • Hal's growing pains remarkably helped in a few
minutes with unusually safe method • Correct diagnosis
of dietary deficiencies is the key to successful treatment
••• How You Can Benefit from the Case Histories in This
Chapter

A practical working definition of folk medicine • A fruit
that miraculously heals arthritis, rheumatism and gout:
six case histories • An astounding new treatment for
stubborn prostate problems • Rectal itching alleviated by
unusually easy-to-use rare treatment • Vince's hay fever
quickly helped by surprisingly different methods • A
marvelous food that can work wonders for a variety of
ailments: four case histories • Marlene's early glaucoma
turned around ••• Benefits You Can Gain from the Case
Histories in This Chapter

problems • Several cases of hay fever whipped by uncommon treatment • Asthma patient quickly helped by
singular treatment • How Everett's shortness of breath
was relieved in extremely short order ••• How You Can
Benefit from the Case Histories in This Chapter

6 How to Rid Yourself of Upper Digestive Tract Problems Permanently with Fantastic Results • 88

How I got fabulous results with canker sores: four case
histories • Phenomenal benefits for Martha's receding
gums surprise dentist • Two other cases show incredible
improvement in diseased gum tissue • How tooth grinding
was stopped in only one night with unusually quick
treatment • Baby's gas pains completely resolved in less
than an hour with outstanding kitchen remedy • How I
solved George's gastritis with an unusual method • How
you can get rid of heartburn using this exceptional procedure • How you can miraculously relieve occasional
gastric distress • How Frank regained his health after
surgery ••• How the Case Histories in This Chapter Can
Benefit You

7 How to Get Rid of Lower Digestive Problems Forever with Strikingly Different and Unique Methods • 101

How Betty quickly and easily resolved her digestive
problems • Ten years of constipation ended for Sarah with
wondrous improvement • How you, too, can get rid of
constipation using my Three-B Program • Diarrhea cured
with startlingly different approach • Sally's ulcerative
colitis incredibly healed with natural foods • Diverticulitis
gives in to new treatment • Miscellaneous conditions
resolved by this fantastic new diet • Rectal itching
eliminated for Larry • Hemorrhoids relieved for Kenneth
with extraordinary treatment ••• Benefits You Can Gain
from the Case Histories in This Chapter

8 How to Alleviate the Aches and Pains of Arthritis and Rheumatism Naturally with Incredible Success • 114

How the arthritis in Katherine's knees was wonderfully
healed • How Bill found complete freedom from his
troublesome shoulder bursitis • Arthritis in hands of
secretary-typist relieved in only four months • Rheumatism
in writer's wrist miraculously cured by pyridoxine •

all hope • Six-year skin rash amazingly disappears at last • Vitamin E oil works wonders in topical skin use • Three case histories show how little-known mineral solves skin problems safely and quickly • Horrible eczema of hands yields to unconventional treatment ••• How You Can Have a Glowing, Youthful and Radiant Complexion with These Easy-to-Use Methods

11   How to Keep Your Heart and Circulation Remarkably Young and Vital • 156

How your cardiovascular system works • How I lowered Joe's blood pressure with this unusually easy-to-use method • Orville's blood pressure improved with this extraordinary method, too • How Joyce got rid of her high blood pressure and regained her health • How I was able to help Lloyd's heart trouble with natural means • How a cardiac invalid was cured by exceptional measures • Mike's heart responds magnificently to different treatment • Rose gets spectacular results with her heart ailment • How I quickly cured Caroline's aching legs • How Arline got rid of her leg cramps with this safe, easy method • Paul's phlebitis responds superbly in only one short week • Bedfast patient recovers in short order with vitamin E • Even Buerger's disease can be cured with unorthodox treatment ••• How You, Too, Can Keep Your Heart and Circulation Young and Vital • How to recognize angina pectoris • How vitamin E can help angina pectoris • How to prevent an attack of coronary thrombosis • How my heart patients have been helped by vitamin E • How mild exercise can help your heart

12   How to Quickly and Easily Correct Your Low Blood Sugar with Drugless Dietary Methods • 172

How low blood sugar can sap your strength and drain your energy • What actually happens in your body when you have low blood sugar • How Ralph quickly conquered his low blood sugar with these unusually easy-to-use methods • What refined white sugar can do to babies and children • How Eddie overcame his lack of energy and regained his health • Effects of sugar on the body in middle and old age • How Eileen got rid of her digestive problems • Other ailments caused by refined white sugar • How Norman got rid of his sour stomach without dangerous alkalizers • How Helen cured her anemia in short

1

How My Extraordinary Methods of Treatment Bring Quick and Marked Relief to Patients with Chronic Ailments

Shortly after I went into professional practice, I found that most patients with chronic ailments come to a chiropractor only as a last resort. Almost all of them had been the drug route before with little or no results, so I realized that medication was not the answer to their health problems. Had it been, none of them would have been in my office for help. I quickly reached the conclusion that conventional orthodox methods would be useless.

I also discovered very soon that vertebral manipulation or chiropractic adjustment alone was not the total answer in most cases. For instance, a factory worker with chronic headaches would never be relieved only by chiropractic adjustments unless he could be transferred from his job as a paint sprayer on an assembly line where he breathed in noxious fumes eight hours a day. Nor would I be able to cure completely, with nothing but spinal manipulation, the aching and crooked back of a mailman who carried a 35 pound sack of mail over his shoulder six to eight hours a day.

I quickly realized that good skeletal structure, rich red blood, healthy muscle tissue and vital body organs were impossible to build or maintain in good health by chiropractic adjustments alone. Good nutrition, along with the proper vitamins, minerals, proteins, fats and natural carbohydrates, was required, as well as the proper physical environment.

21

All this led me to the realization that most chronic diseases my patients had could be cured with specific common and ordinary foods, vitamins, minerals, enzymes and natural herbs — *but only when used in extraordinary and unorthodox ways.*

This book, then, is a compilation and record of dozens and dozens of actual case histories covering a multitude of ailments. Each case is authentic and documented. Of course, the patients' names have all been changed to protect their privacy. Other than that, however, the factual material presented in this book follows each case history to the letter. Now, for the first patient...

How I cleared up Nancy's nervous problem in two short weeks with this amazing new treatment

I doubt seriously if I have ever seen a more nervous or jumpy person than Nancy when she first came to my office. She could not sit back in her chair and relax for a moment. Instead, she sat up on the edge of it, poised like a bird on a tree branch, ready to fly away at the first sign of danger.

She would flinch and start at the slightest sound. Her nerves seemed as raw and jagged as those of the alcoholic or drug addict suffering from withdrawal symptoms. Her hands were never still. She was constantly picking at some part of herself, scratching, rubbing, digging and poking. It seemed absolutely impossible for her to remain completely quiet for even one minute; some part of her body was always in motion. Little wonder she complained of chronic fatigue and nervous exhaustion.

Her face and body showed the physical effects of her nervous condition — she was twenty pounds underweight. Her hands and arms were bony and thin while her face had a drawn and haggard expression. Deep shadows under her eyes and wrinkles in her forehead added ten years or more to her actual physical age.

Nancy told me she had been taking tranquilizers for more than five years. Her previous doctors, as well as her own friends, had suggested to her that her problem was emotional and that she should seek psychiatric care; but even this had not helped her. She said that without taking a tranquilizer every four hours or so, she was barely able to function due to an over-powering sense of anxiety and nervousness. Finally, in desperation Nancy came to me, thinking her condition might somehow be nutritional rather than psychological, even though none of her doctors had ever suggested such a possibility.

My detailed analysis of Nancy's food intake showed her to be extremely deficient in her zinc consumption. This surprised me, for I usually find a calcium and magnesium deficiency in nervous conditions. However, after double-checking to make sure, I got the same answer, so I immediately started Nancy on 30 milligrams of zinc each day.

The results were amazing to both of us. In fact, they were almost like a miracle. In *only two weeks,* Nancy was a completely changed person. She was no longer nervous and jumpy, nor was she startled by sudden noises. She was calm, collected and completely at ease in the presence of other people.

Nancy hasn't taken a tranquilizer for more than six months now. She feels wonderfully well adjusted, and as she told me, "It's great just to feel normal like everyone else."

She is now up to her correct weight, her arms and hands are properly filled out, and her face no longer has that worn and haggard look it once had. In fact, today Nancy appears to be several years younger than her actual age instead of ten years older as she did before.

Nancy still takes her zinc supplement even though she shows no sign of a nervous problem anymore. My second analysis of her dietary intake, which I did at the end of the first month of treatment, showed her to be still mildly deficient in some of the vitamins and other minerals; so she is also taking a multi-vitamin, multi-mineral supplement to help maintain her good health. However, zinc was the primary factor in solving Nancy's nervous problem. It literally gave her back her good health.

How Sam, my mailman, got rid of his blistered feet with my unusually easy-to-use treatment

Sam, my mailman, came to me desperately looking for help. He was suffering horribly from huge blisters on his feet that had developed from a new pair of improperly fitted shoes.

As Sam told me, he had tried every pharmaceutical product on the market he could find, but he had been unable to gain any relief whatever from the pain and discomfort.

When I saw Sam's feet, I was inclined to tell him to give up, go home, and go to bed for a week; but he was so insistent about staying on the job that I decided to try and devise something to give him some kind of relief.

I remembered that a patient of mine, whose job in a garment factory required her to stand all day, had told me she was able to get relief for her sore and aching feet by rubbing them each night with garlic oil. I knew that garlic oil was antiseptic and would not injure Sam's feet, so I decided to try it. I got some natural garlic perles down from my shelf supply, broke open several of them, and massaged the oil into Sam's sore and blistered feet.

The next day when he stopped by with my mail, I massaged his feet again with garlic oil. I was most gratified to find the swelling greatly reduced. Sam said that the pain had practically disappeared. I followed this same procedure for three more days when Sam delivered my mail, for a total of five treatments. At the end of that time, you would never know that Sam's feet had ever bothered him. They were completely healed and back to normal again.

Why my treatment is considered to be unorthodox and unconventional

I can think of several reasons why the methods I use are considered to be unorthodox and unconventional. Take vitamin therapy, for instance. The textbook I studied in college indicated that a vitamin A deficiency would result primarily in the loss of night vision. Yet I have used vitamin A to correct much more than that — acne, sinusitis, and hay fever just to give you three examples.

In school I learned that a deficiency of the B vitamins could cause beri-beri and pellagra. I have never treated a case of either of these, but I have used the B vitamins successfully in cases of skin rash, painful menstruation, vaginal infection and a variety of other conditions.

I was also taught that vitamin C should be used to treat scurvy. I have never handled a true case of scurvy, but I have used vitamin C to relieve asthma, cure the common cold, combat a sore throat, heal an aching back, and clear up a lymphatic gland infection.

Furthermore, my treatment is considered to be unorthodox and unconventional not only because I use vitamins, minerals, natural foods and herbs to treat conditions other than those listed in the textbook, but also because I use them far in excess of what the book describes as the minimum daily requirement.

For example, the current recommended daily allowance by the United States Food and Drug Administration for vitamin A is 5,000 units for the average adult. I have used as much as 20 times that amount to treat skin conditions before I could get favorable results. I have never had a single adverse reaction in one single case.

The recommended daily allowance for vitamin C is only 60 milligrams. I have used 50 to 100 times that amount and more in my treatment of various cases. I have never had a single adverse reaction occur in any of my patients from such massive vitamin C therapy either.

To best understand why there is no bad side effect in such massive vitamin therapy, as there almost always is in drug therapy, you should know that vitamins are not medicine. *Vitamins are food.* But drugs are drugs. That's all there is to that!

During my years in practice, I have also used many minerals, natural foods and herbs in a variety of unorthodox and unconventional ways to cure conditions that would not yield to so-called normal or orthodox medical treatment. I know that as you read the many case histories given in this book, your eyebrows will often go up in surprise at some of the methods I have used. And I can't say I blame you at all. I myself have met few doctors who have successfully used cherries to cure gout, zinc to combat abnormal body odor, yogurt to relieve diarrhea, cranberries to cure a bladder infection, comfrey tea for muscle pain, cinnamon to stop bed wetting, and so on.

All I can say is this: I cannot always prove the methods I use by laboratory or scientific analysis, but I can show you the clinical results I've obtained. And as far as the sick patient is concerned, that's all that really counts. So let me give you some more examples now of my successful unorthodox and extraordinary methods so you can see for yourself the results I get with sick people.

How Anna quickly got rid of her canker sores with my unique procedures

Anna had suffered from painful canker sores for years before she came to see me. She had tried avoiding various foods and drinks, but none of these procedures gave her any permanent results. Her doctor's solution to her problem was to offer only symptomatic relief instead of trying to determine the cause of her condition. When a friend told her of the benefits she'd received in her own case, Anna came to my office.

The inside of Anna's mouth had several huge canker sores the day I examined her; she also had an extremely large ulcerated area on the end of her tongue. Her cankers were all so painful and sore she could scarcely talk, let alone eat or drink. In fact, she said that many times she was able to drink only liquids when her canker sores were so numerous. If you've ever been troubled with them, you'll know exactly the torture Anna was going through — she was absolutely miserable.

My dietary analysis of Anna's food intake showed her to be lacking in the entire vitamin B complex. To resolve this, I put her on an extremely high potency B complex (B-100 from Puritan's Pride) along with some dessicated liver and brewer's yeast tablets, both of which are also rich in all the B vitamins. I had her take these supplements three times a day.

She responded wonderfully to this treatment, and in only three days her mouth was completely free from sores for the first time in more than ten years. As long as Anna continues her vitamin B supplementation, she has no problems at all with canker sores.

By experimentation Anna has been able to somewhat reduce the amount of vitamin B complex, dessicated liver and brewer's yeast she takes each day to prevent her canker sores from returning. However, she still takes all three of them to be sure to get more than enough of all the vitamin B complex she needs.

If Anna does stop taking her supplements altogether, within three or four days she will have one or more canker sores again. She then must triple or quadruple the amount she normally takes for at least three or four days to get rid of the sores again.

Since vitamin B is a food and not a drug, Anna has learned to accept daily supplementation of it in her diet as a normal routine procedure. She's learned the valuable lesson that if vitamins can solve the problem and get you well, they can also prevent recurrence of the same problem and keep you from getting sick again. Vitamin supplementation is the most inexpensive method I know of to keep you well and maintain your good health.

How Frank amazingly eliminated his hemorrhoids without painful surgery in only 48 hours

When Frank came to see me, he had been suffering from hemorrhoids for nearly three months. The pain was terrible. He had been unable to sleep properly or do a full day's work in all that time. He had tried all sorts of medicinal preparations, suppositories, salves, ointments, and the like, as well as hot sitz baths, but none of these had given him more than a few hours of temporary relief. Bowel movements were an absolutely terrifying experience for him, for the pain was excruciating. Frank was ready to submit to surgery, but before doing so, he decided to come see me in a last desperate attempt to avoid an operation.

My dietary analysis of Frank's food intake showed him to be terribly deficient in vitamin C, which was really not at all surprising to me; for Frank was a chain smoker, burning up three to four packs of cigarettes a day. You see, one cigarette will destroy at least 25 milligrams of vitamin C in the body. Now a medium-sized orange at its best has no more than 75 milligrams of vitamin C, so it takes only three cigarettes to completely destroy the value of that orange. In Frank's case, it would have been absolutely impossible for him to get enough vitamin C from natural sources when he smoked from 60 to 80 cigarettes every day.

I started Frank on a vitamin C supplement and had him take 1,500 milligrams four times a day for a total of 6,000 milligrams. Because his vascular condition indicated a capillary breakdown, I also had him take 150 milligrams four times a day for a total of 600 milligrams of the bioflavonoids — rutin, narigin, and hesperidin — which occur in the pulp and white rind of citrus fruits and are associated with vitamin C and found in conjunction with it. The bioflavonoids, often known as vitamin P, augment and amplify the action of vitamin C in the body by promoting healing and benefiting the circulatory system.

Although I expected good results in Frank's case, nevertheless I was absolutely amazed when he called me a few days later. He said that within 48 hours after starting his treatment, all pain had ceased. His hemorrhoids had subsided and almost disappeared. I could hardly believe it myself. It was almost like a miracle to me, for although I have seen some fantastic results take place over the years from using natural healing methods, Frank's case was one of the quickest to respond that I had ever treated.

Margaret's migraine headaches incredibly relieved after 25 years of misery

Margaret had suffered with migraine headaches since she was ten years old. She was 35 when she came to my office and extremely anxious to get some kind of relief for her problem. Her attacks were always accompanied by violent nausea and vomiting and she would be incapacitated for several days at a time before recovering from one of her migraine seizures.

Unfortunately, my dietary analysis of her food intake offered nothing conclusive for me to work with — which does happen occasionally — so I turned to my previous records and case histories in which I had used folk medicine, often gained from my own patients over the years, to see if I could devise some solution for Margaret.

I came across one case history of an old man who had told me he couldn't control his temper unless he took lecithin. Although he had come to me for a different ailment entirely, I remembered how he had told me that lecithin helped to relieve his nervous tension and keep him calm and at ease.

Since Margaret was an extremely nervous person and she felt her migraine attacks were precipitated by severe nervous tension, I rationalized that if lecithin could help a person control his temper (which in itself is a sign of nervous irritation), then it might well help Margaret's nerves too.

So I recommended that she take lecithin capsules three times a day as well as use lecithin granules on her cereals, in meat loaf, hamburger, casseroles, and so on.

Margaret received tremendous relief from her 25 years of migraine attacks. She takes lecithin all the time now to prevent any recurrence of her attacks. When she thinks she feels a headache coming on, she simply increases her lecithin intake, and as a result, the migraine never quite gets there. As Margaret says, she's most grateful for this relief. I'm sure any of you who've suffered with migraine headaches can appreciate the way she feels.

Hal's growing pains remarkably helped in a few minutes with this unusually safe method

Mrs. J. brought her son, Hal, to me when he was nine. Hal was suffering with "growing pains" in the legs and abdomen. He had suffered off and on with severe leg pains since he'd been ten or eleven months old. Mrs. J. had walked the floor with him night after night because of his crying and inability to sleep. At that time, the family doctor suggested only baby aspirin to kill the pain.

When Hal became able to talk and tell his parents exactly where and how he hurt, they took him to several specialists for help. But after seeing two orthopedic doctors and three podiatrists, they gave up. All they got after several complete physical examinations, a dozen X-rays, and a lot of doctors' fees were some expensive specially built shoes, a recommendation for aspirin to kill the pain, and the statement, "Oh, he's probably just got growing pains. He'll get over them when he gets older."

So Mrs. J. decided to find out all she could about Hal's condition on her own. After reading several books about natural healing methods, vitamins and minerals, she brought Hal to me. Having had experience with this kind of condition before, I went right ahead and treated Hal without making a complete analysis of his dietary intake.

Right there in my office I crushed and mixed a half dozen tablets of dolomite into a glass of milk and had Hal drink it. In less than 30 minutes the pains in his legs were completely gone. No other treatment than dolomite has ever been necessary. Hal takes 2,000 milligrams of dolomite in a tablet form every day and has never been bothered with leg pains since then.

Correct diagnosis of dietary deficiencies is the key to successful treatment

You may wonder as you read why some of my patients are cured by one substance while others with apparently the same condition are relieved by an entirely different one altogether. For example, I have had cases of acne that have been completely healed with vitamin A, while others have needed zinc or the vitamin B complex. Still others have been relieved by a combination of all three of these. Simply said, it all depends on which food element or substance is missing as determined by my analysis of the daily dietary intake.

You see, when a patient first comes to me, an extremely detailed history is taken of his or her dietary habits. A record is made of everything that goes into the patient's mouth. Additional data about smoking, drinking, medical drug usage, vitamin consumption, environmental conditions, and so on are taken into consideration too. When I complete my analysis of all this information, I know which food substances are deficient in the diet. I also know when the patient is eating too much of the wrong kinds of food as well.

I make another dietary analysis at the end of 30 days. During that time, the patient keeps track of every single thing he eats or drinks, including the exact amounts. The second analysis is even more accurate than the first; but I have found that in 98 percent of my cases, it will simply confirm the original one. Only about two percent show a substantial difference between the first and second analyses. The difference is usually due to a patient's faulty memory on the first one. The vitamins, minerals, or other food substances I've asked the patient to take as a result of the first analysis are naturally taken into account on the second one.

Sometimes I cannot find a specific dietary deficiency as in the case of Margaret's migraine headaches, although that is extremely rare. Ninety-nine percent of my patients do have a dietary deficiency of some sort that is causing the problem. Of course, in the case of Sam's blistered feet, I did not even make a dietary analysis of his food intake, for it was not appropriate for me to do so.

In cases like these, I turn to other reference material that I have available for treatment of my patients' problems. By keeping an open and inquisitive mind, I have been able to glean a tremendous amount of information from my patients that I can use to successfully treat ailments in my practice.

I have never felt that just because I was the doctor, I could not gain something from my patients about healing methods. I have never believed in playing God. One of the standard questions I have asked every patient who has come into my office since I began practicing back in 1949 is this: "Do you know of any folk remedy, kitchen medicine, or natural healing method that has helped you or some member of your family in the past?" The answers to that question have given me a broader education than I ever received while I was in college.

Incidentally, if you yourself know of some extraordinary or unconventional treatment that has helped you in the past, please write me in care of the publisher and tell me all about it in full detail. I'd be extremely happy to add it to my file of reference material and most grateful to you for telling me about it.

How You Can Benefit from the Case Histories in This Chapter

Nancy's case history clearly shows that a zinc deficiency can be responsible for nervous strain and tension. If you have such a problem, zinc could well be the answer for you. Ten milligrams three times a day for a total of 30 milligrams is usually enough to cure or prevent a zinc deficiency. I have also found zinc to be highly beneficial in treating such other conditions as an enlarged prostate, acne and other skin conditions, circulatory problems in the feet and legs, abnormal body odor, and the common cold.

Physiologically, zinc is one of the constituents of insulin, so it is vital for energy production and the maintenance of normal blood sugar levels. It is found in the male reproductive fluids and is necessary for the healing of wounds and burns. It is found in many of the body enzymes. You might think you don't have a zinc deficiency, and perhaps you don't, but I can tell you this: eight out of every ten Americans do. If you don't take at least 30 milligrams of zinc every day as a food supplement, chances are you're one of those eight.

* * *

If you have canker sores as Anna had and can relieve them with the vitamin B complex as she did, you would get your money's worth and more again out of this book just for this one small section. If you do decide to use this method, it would be wise to use all three sources of vitamin B just as Anna did, especially a high potency B complex such as the *B-100.* These three supplements, the high potency B complex, dessicated liver, and brewer's yeast tablets, should be taken three times a day with your meals.

Your body needs the vitamin B complex on a daily basis. Don't worry about taking too much of it. Vitamin B is non-toxic and cannot hurt you, no matter how much you take. Any excess in your body is simply passed out in the urine since it is water soluble.

* * *

If you have hemorrhoids as Frank had, an inexpensive way to find out if they can be reduced or eliminated without needless and painful surgery would be to take vitamin C. I would suggest 750 to 1,500 milligrams four times a day for a total of 3,000 to 6,000 milligrams along with a total of 600 milligrams of the bioflavonoids spread out the same way. The only possible side effect from vitamin C is occasional mild diarrhea when too much is taken. To keep this from happening, you could start with a daily total of 1,500 or 2,000 milligrams and slowly increase your intake each day.

I have also found that hemorrhoidal pain is much worse in heavy coffee drinkers. If you have that habit, try limiting your coffee intake to one cup at breakfast. That action in itself is often enough to bring marked relief to a hemorrhoid sufferer.

* * *

If you suffer from migraines as Margaret did, I'm sure you'll agree that lecithin is worth a try. How much you should take is a hard question to answer since I don't know your individual circumstances. If I were you, I would use both capsules and granules as Margaret did. You can start with the amount recommended by the maker for each of these. If you don't get results with that, double those amounts. If need be, triple or quadruple your intake until you do get results. As with all other food supplements, lecithin is a food. It is non-toxic. It cannot harm you, and, in fact, it will always help you.

You'll gain another tremendous benefit by using lecithin if you're troubled with a high cholesterol level. One of the best ways to prevent cholesterol deposits in the blood vascular system is not to consume less cholesterol in the diet, but to consume more lecithin. Its presence in the blood stream helps to keep the blood cholesterol in solution and to dissolve cholesterol deposits that have already formed.

* * *

Dolomite is a truly magical food for "growing pains." As you saw, Hal "outgrew" his growing pains in less than 30 minutes in my office. He didn't have to wait until he got older.

If you have growing children who suffer from leg cramps or abdominal pains, you don't need a dietary analysis to find out what's wrong with them. They need more calcium in the form of dolomite, so don't let some doctor tell you they have growing pains that will disappear when they get older. That's not true, and here's why:

It just isn't normal for the body to have pain. It isn't built that way. Whenever there is pain, there has to be a good rea-

son for it. Dolomite with its calcium and magnesium is the answer to growing pains. It can also solve the problem of cramping painful menstruation that occurs so often in the teens. And if you're suffering from leg cramps, especially in the calves of your legs at night, you could probably use some extra dolomite too, just like your children.

How much dolomite should you take? Enough to get results. I have found that approximately 2,000 milligrams a day is required by the average patient who needs extra calcium. However, with older people, overweight people, as well as those who are anemic, excitable, nervous or depressed, I have used as much as 4,000 and 5,000 milligrams a day to get results. Calcium is often poorly absorbed and assimilated by the body, so these higher amounts are sometimes necessary.

You need not be at all concerned about the amount you take, for there is no possibility whatever of any danger due to an excess of dolomite. The calcium-magnesium combination found in dolomite is safe in any conceivable supplement quantity. I always use dolomite instead of bonemeal since bonemeal contains phosphorus. It is almost never necessary to take additional phosphorous because it is generally well supplied in the average diet. In fact, I cannot remember a case where I've ever found a phosphorus deficiency. Too much phosphorus causes the body to excrete calcium and is often the reason for a calcium deficiency. That's why dolomite is so much better to use.

2

Uncommon Folk Remedies I've Used That Really Work to Make You Well

A practical working definition of folk medicine

From my own point of view, I feel that a food or a food substance, according to my definition of a folk remedy, must meet these three criteria:

1. *It must be readily available.* You should be able to find it in your average large supermarket or health food store. If an item that you read about cannot be obtained easily, there's very little use of you even learning about it or how it works or what it does.

This has been one of my pet peeves about most folk medicine books I've read before. They specify some exotic foreign plant or root from the Orient which I cannot find since I do not have a San Francisco Chinatown or a Japanese grocery store around the corner. As a result, the information is virtually useless to me. I have not included one single item in this book that you cannot find in your grocery store, your supermarket or your health food store — no matter where you live.

2. *It should not be a prescription drug or a controlled medicine.* If it falls in this category, if your family physician has to write a prescription before you can get the item, then it is not readily available and cannot possibly be considered to be a folk remedy or a kitchen medicine.

3. *It must actually work to make you well.* I have seen

some substances included in folk medicine books that offered no documentary proof of their efficacy. I dislike and mistrust statements that read, "It has been reported that..." To me, this is not proof; this is a copout. As far as I am concerned, "It has been reported that" falls into the same category as "They said," a statement that used to drive me up the wall when I was in the service away back when. I want proof — not fairy tales or rumor.

Every food substance in this book is documented by a factual case history. Either I have used it myself on my own patients, or as you will find in Chapter 4, I have received first-hand reports from patients who have successfully used such remedies on themselves. Every single case reported to me by a patient has also been documented or verified by some member of the family to serve as an eyewitness. In most of the cases that have been reported to me, I have personally seen the results myself. An eyewitness takes it out of the "They said," "It has been reported that," or "Hear-say" category.

A fruit that miraculously relieves arthritis, rheumatism and gout: six case histories

Shortly after I went into practice, one of my patients, the hard working wife of a farmer, answered my standard question about any folk remedy or kitchen medicine that had helped either her or a member of her family by saying she had rheumatism at one time and cured it by eating cherries. I jotted the information down and filed it away for future use. It was not long before I had the chance to try this new folk remedy. The woman who hobbled through the door a week later was the first of many such cases. I want to tell you about just six of them.

1. *Sore stiff knees helped by cherries.* Ethyl had been suffering with aching throbbing knees for nearly two years. She had already been to several medical specialists, an osteopath, and two chiropractors without obtaining any favorable results. She was taking aspirin constantly to help kill the worst of the pain. Ethyl was only 31 years old. With three children to take care of, she was ready to do almost anything to get some kind of relief.

I told Ethyl about the farmer's wife who had cured her rheumatism by eating cherries and asked her if she'd like to at least try her remedy to see what would happen. She agreed to do so and on the way home she bought several cans of cherries. She ate a bowl of them every day. At the end of one week, the pain, swelling and stiffness in her knees were all completely gone. As Ethyl told me later, it was almost as if a miracle had taken place.

As long as Ethyl eats some cherries every day, she suffers no pain whatever. She does her housework, walks, exercises, bicycles and bowls, all without pain. Last year during the busy rush and confusion of the holiday season, she forgot all about her daily bowl of cherries. The week after Christmas her knees swelled up, became stiff again, and she suffered severe pain. She went straight to the store and bought 12 cans of cherries: one week later, all the symptoms had disappeared. As Ethyl told me, "Once in a while I get tired of eating cherries every day, but it's really a small price to pay for freedom from pain."

2. *Bert's gout cured by dark sweet cherries.* Bert regards his recovery from gout as a wonderful miracle, too. He had gout in his big toe on the right foot when he came to see me. He was suffering intense pain in the ball of the big toe which was red, hot, swollen, shiny and so sensitive that he could not stand even the slightest pressure. He could not wear a sock or shoe, nor could he stand the touch of a bed sheet on his foot at night. No pain killer or drug had brought him any relief whatever.

I knew of no chiropractic spinal adjustment that would help Bert. I told him about cherries, and although he was doubtful about them being able to help, he figured he had nothing to lose but his gout. So he agreed at least to give them a try.

On the morning of the third day, a Monday, he walked into my office smiling and happy. He had eaten nothing but dark sweet cherries since late Friday afternoon. In only a little over two days — from Friday night until Monday morning — they not only gave him complete relief from the gout in his big toe, but they also helped the rheumatism in his shoulders and back.

3. *Lucy's stiff fingers helped by cherries.* Lucy was 63 years old, had never had an operation, and was in reasonably good health when she came to see me. However, she was suffering from arthritis in her hands and fingers.

I asked her to try cherries which had been so successful for me in other cases of arthritis and rheumatism and she agreed to do so, although as she told me later, she was disappointed at being given such a simple remedy. She had expected me to use some mysterious exotic substance to cure her arthritis.

Lucy ate a bowl of cherries and drank the juice every day faithfully for two weeks. At the end of that time, she found there was a tremendous improvement in her fingers. The swelling was much less than before and the pain was gone completely. She is now able to make a fist for the first time in many years.

4. *Norma's rheumatism helped by cherries.* Norma also suffered from rheumatism in her hands and fingers. They were swollen, painful, and so stiff she could hardly pick up anything with them. She could not even hold a pen or pencil to write a letter.

A week after she started on her daily consumption of cherries, she woke up one morning to find she felt like a brand-new person. The skin on her hands was clear, the swelling was gone, and she could bend her fingers completely without pain.

Even her wrists and ankles were slimmer than before. This surprised her, for she had not even realized that they were swollen. As Norma told me, "Painful years of suffering and unsightly, cracked, sometimes even bleeding hands were gone. I just can't believe yet a bowl of cherries could do that for me."

5. *Arthritis helped by cherries in only a few hours.* In November, Sue came to me for arthritis in her left arm and shoulder. When I suggested she try cherries to relieve the pain, she refused to believe they could help and left my office in disgust.

I didn't hear from Sue until February the next year. After she left my office in November, she simply decided not to follow my advice, nor did she go to another doctor. She tried to get along on aspirin and "tough it out" as she said, for she was tired of going to doctors and not getting any results. She had a miserable winter, taking aspirin almost by the handful, soaking in a hot tub, using a heating pad trying to kill the pain — but all to no avail.

In February her son wanted her to bake a cherry pie for Washington's birthday. While Sue was working in the kitchen baking the pie, she remembered what I had told her about cherries for the pains of arthritis and rheumatism. She suddenly decided to try them. She opened another can of cherries, sat down at her kitchen table, and ate them all. Then she got up and went about her work.

A few hours later, it suddenly dawned on Sue that all the pain had vanished from her arm and shoulder for the first time she could remember in years. As she told me in my office later, "It was too good to be true, Doctor. I can hardly believe it even yet."

She still eats cherries every day and her problem has never returned. Her family laughs at her and tells her she's crazy, that cherries can't help arthritis or rheumatism. But Sue lets them laugh all they want to; she keeps right on eating cherries anyway.

I tell her not to worry about it. Poeple have laughed at me many times before, too, for my unorthodox methods and unconventional treatment. It doesn't bother me one bit. I'm happy to see sick people get well by using my extraordinary methods.

6. *Gout cured by cherries.* Keith had been suffering from gout for a long time. The medication he was taking had helped the pain somewhat, but the swelling had not subsided. In fact, it slowly got worse and spread up to his ankle which caused pain to radiate up into the calf of his leg.

Keith's recovery was not as dramatic as Bert's was; but after all, he had had the gout much, much longer. He decided to give the cherry therapy a try. In the end it was successful, though it did take two months to get the results we wanted.

At the end of that time, the swelling was completely gone and he had greatly reduced his medication to kill the pain. By the end of the third month, Keith was able to dispense with his medication altogether. He has continued to eat cherries every day, and he has never had a recurrence of any of his symptoms in the past year.

An astounding new treatment for stubborn prostate problems

Neal was suffering from a swollen prostrate gland when he came to see me. It was extremely difficult for him to urinate and it took a long time for him to get the stream started. There was also a decrease in the force of the urinary stream and it was much smaller in diameter than before. As a result, the bladder was not being completely voided, and Neal found himself trying to urinate every 15 minutes or so. But he could void only a small amount each time, usually ending up just dribbling a few drops. Neal was getting up a dozen times at night to go to the bathroom. He was suffering from pain in the lower abdomen over the bladder region which was especially noticeable upon palpation. He had a constant dull ache across the small of his back.

Neal had consulted with a urologist before coming to see me. This doctor had recommended removal of the prostate gland. That is actually why Neal came to me: he wanted to try something first that was not as drastic as an operation.

One of my patients had told me how he recovered from prostate trouble by eating six bee pollen tablets a day, so I recommended the same procedure to Neal. In two weeks his symptoms had lessened considerably. At the end of one month, they were gone altogether. Neal's urologist examined him again and told him that although he still had some benign enlargement of his prostate, it was now not enough to warrant surgical intervention, especially since all his previous symptoms had mysteriously subsided.

Neal had continued to have a check-up every six months by his urologist. Even though two years have now gone by, he has not had to take any further action. He still takes six bee pollen tablets every day. Neal is 71 years old. He walks a couple of miles each day and seems to be in perfect health, much different than when he first came to see me.

Rectal itching alleviated by unusually easy-to-use rare treatment

Sid told me he had scratched his rump for more than ten years. It itched constantly and was a source of embarrassment to him since he couldn't keep his hands off it. He scratched himself all the time. Doctors had told him it was caused by the use of antibiotics that had killed off the friendly bacteria in his digestive tract. He had tried various foods normally helpful in re-establishing the proper intestinal flora such as yogurt and buttermilk, but the constant itching still persisted. Salves and ointments seemed only to compound the problem rather than help it.

Analysis of Sid's dietary intake showed a high deficiency in vitamin E. I placed him on a high potency supplement of mixed tocopherols — 200 units three times daily for a total of 600 units — to build up the vitamin E reserves in his body.

Then, since wheat germ oil also contains vitamin E, I asked Sid to apply it several times a day to the affected area, making sure it was thoroughly cleansed first. It's been three weeks now since he first came to me. He's had no sign of an itch since. The sores created by scratching and digging have all healed up. As Sid puts it, "Only someone who has scratched his rear end for as long as I have can appreciate what a relief this is."

Vince's hay fever quickly helped by surprisingly different methods

Vince came to my office for a completely unrelated problem that had nothing to do with hay fever. But during the course of taking his past history, he told me he had suffered with hay fever for many years.

A patient of mine had told me she used to suffer with hay fever — until she learned the value of raw honey. She takes two tablespoons of raw honey a day, starting about six weeks before hay fever time. She continues to take it until the season is over. She has not been troubled with hay fever for the past five or six years.

Vince agreed that it was worth a try, for he'd always had to take shots before and stay in an air conditioned office or house all during the hay fever season. Honey really worked wonders for him. This is his second year now without shots and he no longer is a prisoner of air conditioning. He goes outside whenever he wants to and has no sign of his former problem.

Vince's son also suffered from hay fever. The first year he refused to try the honey because he didn't like the taste of it, so he stuck with the shots. But when he saw the wonderful results in his father's case, he decided to try the honey therapy, too. Not once has he had to resort to shots since he started using it. Raw honey has solved his hay fever problem, too.

A marvelous food that can work wonders for a variety of ailments: four case histories

Although my mother and my wife both have always used garlic in their cooking, it was not until I got into practice that I found out from several of my patients how to use it as a healing agent as well as a food. Even though I have used it now for many years successfully in my practice, I never cease to be amazed at its versatility. You'll see these diverse qualities of garlic for yourself as you read the following case histories.

1. *Janet's impetigo cured by garlic oil.* Janet came to me suffering with impetigo on her hands and face. She was horribly embarrassed by her appearance and willing to do anything to get rid of her ugly lesions and the itching. She had already undergone several weeks of treatment by a dermatologist who had used various salves and ointments without any success.

I cleansed Janet's hands and face thoroughly with soap and water and then rubbed some garlic oil on the lesions. I also had her take two garlic perles internally. Then I asked her to wait in one of the dressing rooms while I attended to some other patients.

An hour later when I returned to see her, the itching had completely subsided. The wild harassed look in her eyes was gone. I gave her some garlic oil capsules and told her to take two of them with every meal. I also asked her to open some of the capsules and rub the oil into the skin of her hands and face at least three times daily. No other treatment was used.

That night Janet was able to sleep comfortably without scratching for the first time in three weeks and more. She continued her garlic oil treatment and in only three short days her infectious impetigo was completely gone.

2. *Floyd's stomach distress and chronic diarrhea relieved by garlic.* Floyd suffered constantly from indigestion along with chronic diarrhea. Analysis of his dietary intake proved to be negative, so I was at somewhat of a loss as to how to proceed. As usual, I turned to my files on folk remedies and kitchen medicines. I found that garlic was often beneficial in cases of stomach distress with an unknown cause.

Floyd agreed to try some garlic capsules for his condition. He began taking six a day — two with each meal — and almost miraculously, his stomach problem was solved a couple of days later. About a week after that, his chronic diarrhea stopped. It has not returned now for more than three months, nor has he had any more trouble with his stomach.

Floyd also received a side benefit from the garlic: when I examined him initially, I found his blood pressure to be quite elevated, 190 over 110. But upon examining him again a few days ago, I found his pressure was down to 140 over 90, a perfectly acceptable figure for his age. In fact, I've had far younger patients than Floyd with much higher blood pressure reading than that.

3. *Kenneth's bedsores helped by garlic oil.* An elderly patient of mine, Kenneth, fell and broke his hip. His regular medical doctor set it and Kenneth was confined to bed, waiting for it to heal properly. During that time he developed a bedsore, and his wife, Doris, called me to help.

I took some garlic oil capsules to their house with me, opened some of them, and rubbed the oil gently into Kenneth's sore. He said it burned and smarted a little but other than that, it didn't bother him. I told Doris to put a loose bandage over it so it could get plenty of air but still be protected.

When she took the bandage off the next morning she noticed the swelling was down and the bedsore looked much better. She rubbed some more garlic oil on it and placed another loose bandage over it.

The second morning when Doris removed the bandage she found the scab had fallen off, the swelling was completely gone, and there was no bleeding whatever. The skin had a healthy pink appearance.

Doris continued to massage the area daily with garlic oil for a week. All the dead skin around the opening peeled off and left the skin smooth and clear. Kenneth had no further trouble.

4. *Skin infection cured by garlic.* One of my patients, Lewis, felt a rough spot on his chin. Without realizing it, he kept rubbing and pecking at it. It turned red, itched, and began to spread. He thought he had some kind of fungus infection, so he put a great deal of a fungus ointment on it. This only made it worse. It would form a hard crust and become red and rough again.

He thought of going to a dermatologist, but since he was already a patient of mine for another ailment, he decided to come to me. I took some garlic oil capsules, cut them open, and rubbed some of the garlic oil on the infected area. I gave Lewis some to take along and told him to take at least six capsules a day orally and to keep the area on his chin constantly anointed with garlic oil. In three days Lewis called me to report that the eruption had disappeared completely. The area was back to normal again.

Marlene's early glaucoma turned around

In August Marlene had a glaucoma test by her optometrist. The pressure was 35 in one eye and 33 in the other. Although she was only 35, the doctor suspected early glaucoma.

Marlene's eye doctor used drops, but they did not reduce the pressure; they also irritated her eyes. Then he suggested they try some stronger drops, but she refused. However, Marlene did agree to come back for another glaucoma test six months later in January.

In October Marlene came to me with a bad cold. She felt extremely worn out and run down and dreaded the coming winter. She said she usually got a cold in the fall and couldn't get rid of it until the following spring.

My dietary analysis showed Marlene to be extremely low in her vitamin C intake, so I put her on 6,000 milligrams of vitamin C each day — 2,000 milligrams with each meal — along with 150 milligrams of the bioflavonoids spread out the same way.

Marlene continued to come in on a monthly basis for a check-up. For the first time in many years she did not suffer with a winter cold. When she came in for her February check-up, she had some most interesting news to tell me. She'd been back to her optometrist in January to have her glaucoma test run again. Amazingly, her eye pressures were perfectly normal. Her eye doctor was amazed. He could hardly believe it. In fact, he ran the tests several times to make absolutely sure.

Benefits You Can Gain from the
Case Histories in This Chapter

If you have problems with arthritis, rheumatism or gout, I know of no more inexpensive remedy than cherries. It does not really matter what kind you use: the sour red variety or the sweet dark kind. I've seen patients recover with either one or both. One can a day should be enough to bring relief. If the cherry therapy doesn't appeal to you, then turn to Chapter 8 for some more folk remedies that can be helpful to your arthritis or your rheumatism.

* * *

If you suffer from prostate problems such as a simple non-malignant enlargement, you might find half a dozen bee pollen tablets a day will do the job for you instead of painful surgical removal. Other doctors have found bee pollen tablets to be useful in prostate problems, too. A one-year study of nine patients with prostate problems conducted by Professor G.W. Heise of the Magdeburg Academy of Medicine revealed that all the patients responded to bee pollen treatment with definite improvement.

I do not know what active element in bee pollen causes the improvement. It could be the magnesium or the zinc, both of which are grossly deficient in the average American diet today. It also might be worth noting that prostatic enlargement, which is extremely common today, was rare before 1900. In fact, it

was often regarded as a pathological curiosity. I am only specu-
lating, but when honey used to be the sweetener the average
family used, enlarged prostates were uncommon. Today, enlarged prostates are found in 76 percent of all men over 55,
and white refined sugar is used in almost every home instead
of honey. Bee pollen and honey go together, so there must be
a connection there somewhere.

* * *

Wheat germ oil is a soothing oil to use on various skin
lesions. The vitamin E content helps to heal the infected area.
One of the skin problems I've seen so often in recent years in
teenagers is a rectal itching and inflammation that is caused by
wearing blue jeans without underclothing. The dye in the jeans
is evidently the skin irritant that causes the inflammation and
infection. Wheat germ oil and undershorts correct this problem
immediately.

* * *

Hay fever is such a nuisance to so many people. If you
suffer with it, use honey yourself, a couple of tablespoons every
day. Use it in place of sugar. I use it in my tea all the time. Even
if you don't get rid of your hay fever with honey, your health
will improve; for honey is nature's food, a natural carbohydrate, not a manufactured chemical substance like sugar. Honey
is good for many other conditions, too. Just for instance, it will
calm your nerves and help you get a good night's restful sleep.

* * *

You can use garlic oil on almost all skin lesions with great
success. It is antiseptic and soothing and tends to heal infections quite rapidly just as it did in the case of Janet's impetigo.
Or if you have stomach distress, intestinal problems, even
diarrhea, garlic may well be the solution for you just as it was
for Floyd. Two capsules with each meal would be appropriate
to take.

It is much easier to prevent a bedsore than to heal one. If
you have someone in your family who is confined to bed, constantly change his or her position to prevent bedsores from
developing. Massage is also beneficial as a preventive measure.
If a bedsore does develop, you can use garlic oil to help heal it.

I would recommend that you not give up too soon on any home remedy for any disease you have, no matter what it is. One of our American faults is wanting everything done yesterday, if not sooner.

But you cannot expect that when you're dealing with the human body. Perhaps you might be fortunate and get results in a couple of days as Bert did; and again it might take two or three months to get the desired results as in Keith's case.

I have learned that a good rule of thumb to use for determining how long you should continue your treatment is this: *it takes approximately one month of treatment for every year a person has been sick to get the desired or the maximum results.* Of course, this does not always hold true in every case since there will always be those exceptions, but it is a good general guideline to use.

I do want to make something quite clear at this point: I am not advocating home treatment or folk remedies for a lump in the breast, a sore that fails to heal, a constant cough, a prostate that is nodular, or for any other ailment that might turn out to be cancerous. The best thing for you to do is to get cancer ruled out first by your doctor.

But if all he can do for you, after he's ruled out cancer, is give you some drug to help kill the pain, you are perfectly justified to turn to folk medicine or any other unorthodox treatment to get relief, no matter how long it takes or what has to be done. After all, you're the one with the pain — not your doctor.

3

Unusual Health Problems I've Been Able to Quickly Solve with My Extraordinary Yet Easy-to-Use Treatment

A great many times a patient receives several fringe benefits from using natural foods, vitamins and minerals instead of drugs to cure his ailment. First of all, there are no bad side effects as there usually are with drugs. Second, the use of natural foods, vitamins and minerals to cure a deficiency disease — which most chronic conditions are — goes right to the cause of the ailment. This is not symptomatic treatment as is so often the case in the use of drugs. Third, when the patient's dietary intake is restored to normal, he often finds that other problems besides the major complaint are resolved, too. The first case history is a specific example of that.

Unusual treatment restores the sense of smell for Barry

Barry came to me for help with his sex life. He was in his late fifties and as he told me, he had lost almost all interest in sexual relations with his wife. Once a month was about it, and even then he had difficulty maintaining an erection long enough to reach a satisfactory climax.

Barry's physical examination revealed a uniform enlargement of the prostate gland. I immediately assumed his sexual problem could be the result of a zinc shortage, for a low zinc intake almost always means an enlarged prostate. Not only that, zinc is one of the elements found in the male reproductive fluids; it is vital to normal sexual function. Dietary analysis of Barry's food intake confirmed my original suspicions. He was not getting enough zinc.

I had Barry take 30 milligrams of zinc — 10 milligrams three times a day — and before the first month had gone by, he and his wife were enjoying normal sexual relationships again. Now that I've told you about the primary complaint, let me tell you about the other benefits Barry gained from his zinc therapy.

Barry's sinuses had bothered him for a great many years. In fact, as he told me later, he had lost his sense of smell about five years before. A couple of months after he was on the zinc therapy, he noticed his food seemed much tastier than previously.

Next Barry noticed he was not having as much sinus drainage as before and there seemed to be less mucus formation. One night as he was sitting on his front porch he smelled a skunk. Then it dawned on him what had happened. He had regained his sense of smell that had been lost for so long.

This came as an extremely pleasant surprise to Barry, and to me too. Gaining fringe benefits happens so often with my patients that I really should be prepared for them by now and accept them as a matter of course, but I've never been quite able to do so. I'm always thrilled and overjoyed when this happens.

How we whipped Beulah's bad breath

Beulah had suffered from bad breath and a horrible taste in her mouth for more than ten years. She had tried all sorts of mouth washes and had regular dental check-ups, but nothing seemed to help her at all.

When I analyzed Beulah's dietary intake, I found her to be extremely deficient in one of the vitamins of the B complex, specifically *niacin*. I gave her a high potency vitamin B complex containing all the B vitamins and an additional supplement of *nicotinic acid* specifically to combat her niacin shortage.

Although the primary deficiency indicated by my dietary analysis was niacin, I gave Beulah the entire B complex along with the supplement of nicotinic acid since it is always better to use the B vitamins in their entirety rather than just individually.

Beulah has faithfully taken her vitamin B supplements for two months now, and her extremely bad breath has finally disappeared after all these years. She has found, though, that if she does not take her vitamins on a daily basis, her problem soon reappears.

How Jerry got rid of his backache as if by magic

Jerry was my regular letter carrier before he retired and Sam took his place. At that time I was practicing in Missouri. Winters in the midwest can be miserable for a mailman, and Jerry seemed especially susceptible to colds and respiratory infections. As he told me, "I get a cold in November and I hack and cough and sniffle until late April or early May."

One fall Jerry came to me to see if I could somehow get him through the winter without his catching a bad cold. Dietary analysis showed him to be terribly deficient in vitamin C. I put him on 6,000 milligrams of vitamin C daily — 1,500 milligrams four times a day. I also supplemented the vitamin C with 200 milligrams of bioflavonoids — 50 milligrams four times a day. The end result was that Jerry made it through the winter without a cold for the first time in nearly 15 years.

But as wonderful as this was, there was a fringe benefit that was also quite interesting. Jerry had suffered with low back pain for as long as he could remember. He had tried everything he could think of: massage, heating pads, soft mattresses, hard mattresses and so on, but he still had his nagging backache. He blamed it on his occupation and carrying a heavy bag of mail that made him walk lopsided 30 hours or so every week.

He had not mentioned his low back problem when he first came to see me, for he was primarily interested in avoiding a winter cold. But after he'd been taking vitamin C and the bioflavonoids for about two months, he told me his backache had disappeared for the first time since he'd started carrying mail.

When spring came and the winter cold and flu season was over, Jerry decided to experiment. He stopped taking his vitamin C supplements. His backache returned. When he started taking them again, his backache went away. As you can no doubt guess, Jerry still takes a vitamin C supplement all the time. I now recommend additional vitamin C for all my patients who come to me with low back problems. It has worked wonders for them.

How Karen's menstrual problems improved with natural methods

Karen came to me to see if I could help her get over her extremely painful and heavy menstrual periods. She was 28 years old and had been troubled with her periods since she was 16.

During the past year Karen had been taking aspirin in heavy doses to try and relieve the pain. When her period started, she would take two or three aspirin at once. Then, if that did not help relieve the pain in an hour or so, she would take four or five more. She kept this up until the pain stopped. This procedure continued during her entire menstrual period. She was consuming close to a bottle of aspirin in six or seven days.

Her bleeding was almost hemorrhagic in nature, but Karen did not realize that aspirin was mainly responsible. Aspirin in the quantities she was taking slows the clotting of blood by preventing platelet aggregation, thus causing severe and profuse bleeding.

Karen's dietary intake was deficient in almost all the vitamins and minerals, but she was especially lacking in calcium. Since calcium is also important and necessary for the proper clotting of blood, I gave her 15 dolomite tablets right there in my office. Within 30 minutes the pain stopped. An hour later, I gave her another 15 tablets. An hour after that, her blood flow had slowed down and become minimal.

I also placed Karen on a multi-vitamin, multi-mineral supplement with plenty of iron to build up her blood and let her gain back her strength. She was just on the verge of a severe chronic anemia from all the blood loss during her menstrual periods.

In addition to her other vitamins and minerals, Karen continues to take 2,000 milligrams of calcium every day in the form of dolomite. She has never again suffered a heavy painful menstrual flow. Her periods are now quite normal, painless, and of short duration.

Esther's severe vaginal infection completely healed with this extraordinary procedure

Esther had developed a severe vaginal infection that bothered her for close to a year. It caused intense itching and inflammation and interfered greatly with her normal sex life. A gynecologist had given her a prescription for vaginal suppositories to cure the infection. She used the first prescription for three months. When this failed to produce the desired results, her doctor gave her another prescription which she used for another three months. Her problem still persisted, for even though the second medication brought her some temporary relief, especially from the itching, as soon as she stopped taking it the infection would come back.

Finally, Esther and her husband decided that her ailment might somehow be the result of a nutritional problem, for they simply had run out of other things to blame it on. So Esther came to see me, although with some hesitation, feeling that the idea of a nutritional cause for her vaginal infection was too farfetched.

However, she felt better when I told her that all sorts of conditions in the human body can come from not getting the right kinds of food. The sexual reproductive system is no exception and it is just as vulnerable to ailments caused by nutritional deficiencies as is the digestive system, the cardiovascular system, or the bones and joints, muscles and nerves, and so on.

My analysis of Esther's dietary intake showed that she was extremely deficient in the entire complex of the B vitamins. I had her take a high potency B complex, some dessicated liver, and brewer's yeast tablets four times a day to make sure I had covered every possible vitamin B deficiency.

In only two days the itching stopped and the inflammation subsided. Esther has continued to take her vitamin B supplements and her condition has not come back at all during the past three months. If she stops taking her vitamins, it is possible her vaginitis might return; but as I tell her, taking vitamins is not the same as taking medication. Vitamins are food; medicines are not.

Armond's chronic lymphatic gland infection
finally cured with fabulous results

Armond had been suffering off and on for several years with periodic infections of his lymph glands. Doctors had brushed him aside with such comments as "You'll get over it ...it'll go away...you'll just have to learn to live with it," and the like. None of them had ever taken his condition seriously.

When Armond came to see me, he was in the midst of one of his infectious periods. The glands in his neck and under his jaw were swollen, tender to touch, and extremely hot. I suspected a smoldering infection in his throat or sinuses from this.

I found that Armond was highly deficient in his vitamin C intake, so I immediately placed him on 8,000 milligrams — 2,000 milligrams four times a day. Within less than a week, the swollen lymph glands had reduced in size until they were just barely palpable. They were no longer hot or painful to the touch.

After the initial recovery from his infection, I reduced Armond's daily vitamin C intake down to 4,000 milligrams — 1,000 milligrams four times a day — to prevent any recurrences of his infection. He has not been bothered with the problem now for more than 18 months.

How Gladys gained wonderful relief from
her troublesome hot flashes

Around her 45th birthday, Gladys began to experience all those unmistakable signs of the change of life. Her menstrual periods became irregular. She suffered miserably from hot flashes, which came every few minutes, 30 to 40 times a day. They became almost unbearable for they would be accompanied by profuse sweating, dizziness and fatigue. These hot flashes would then be followed by chills, a rapid pulse, and palpitation of the heart. Her hands and feet would tingle and become numb.

She wanted to see if she could correct her condition by natural methods rather than by using artificial hormone therapy so she came to see me. I found that Gladys was woefully deficient in vitamin E. I started her on 1,200 units a day, 400 at each meal. After only one week of treatment, her hot flashes disappeared altogether. Gladys was very happy, for this had been her major complaint. Her menstrual periods soon became regular and normal once more.

After the hot flashes disappeared, I slowly reduced her vitamin E intake. Gladys is now taking 300 units a day, 100 with each meal. She will continue to do so although she has had no recurrence of her problem in the last 15 months.

How Dorothy is able to control
cystic mastitis by natural means

Two years ago, Dorothy was diagnosed as having chronic cystic mastitis (breast cysts). She suffered a lot of pain and premenstrual discomfort in her breasts. At those times the cysts were extremely tender and could be easily palpated.

Her doctor first recommended surgery, but Dorothy refused. Then he suggested hormone therapy, but she did not want that kind of treatment either. Since her doctor assured her the cysts were not cancerous, she decided to live with her problem and make the best of it.

However, after a while she again grew dissatisfied with her condition and came to see me. I examined her and determined that she needed some additional calcium and magnesium. I had her take 20 tablets of dolomite a day (which gave her 2,600 milligrams of calcium and 1,200 milligrams of magnesium) with wonderful results.

The dolomite causes the cysts to decrease in size, and they almost disappear between her menstrual periods. She no longer suffers any pain or discomfort, nor are the cysts tender to touch as they once were during her menstrual periods. They do not disappear entirely, for during each menstruation they enlarge slightly, but they are not uncomfortable to her at all any more.

But if Dorothy forgets to take her dolomite daily, her next menstrual period is extremely difficult for her. She suffers excessive pain, tenderness and swelling in both breasts. But just as soon as she starts taking her dolomite again, the pain and swelling go away.

I am at a complete loss to explain the physiology of this case. All I can do is report the facts of the case history to you as they are, and that is what I have done.

Troublesome poison ivy healed with new and different method

Gary came to me with a case of poison ivy last spring. This kind of case is really out of my line because I leave surgery, fractures, injuries and poisons to the medical doctors; but since Gary was one of my regular patients, I wanted to help him. Besides, he told me when he'd used commercial drug store preparations before, it took him nearly six weeks to get over the problem.

After studying some case histories and other records, I decided to use vitamin E on his poison ivy. I have some vitamin E capsules with little tits on the end that can be cut off so the oil runs out and can be used externally. I got a couple of these and applied the vitamin E oil to Gary's poison ivy rash.

Then I gave him some more capsules to take along and told him to use the same procedure several times a day. I also asked him to keep me informed as to his progress.

The first thing Gary noticed after applying the vitamin E was that the rash did not spread any further as it had done when he had it previously. The itching and discomfort eased almost at once and then stopped completely 24 hours later. After only five days of treatment — during which time he suffered no discomfort whatever — all Gary could see were a few spots that were rapidly fading away.

Laura's menstrual problems quickly resolved with unusually safe procedure

Laura came to me after talking to Karen. When Karen told her how I had helped with her menstrual problems, Laura called me immediately for an appointment.

Laura told me she was the witch of all witches from a week before her period was due until it was over. Her husband hated to come home from work and would even volunteer to work overtime when she was like this. She said she would scream her head off at her children for minor things and then get so depressed for doing so that she would hate herself.

I assured Laura she wasn't a witch at all, but that chances were some vital food factor was missing from her diet that was making her nervous and causing her to act like one. Sure enough, I found her to be highly deficient in the vitamin B complex.

As soon as this supplement was added to her diet, she was no longer bothered by her periods. She became an angel to her family instead of a witch. Her husband was so grateful he called to thank me for restoring peace and harmony to their family life.

How the Case Histories in This Chapter Can Benefit You

Although a zinc deficiency is not the only cause of sexual incapacity in the male, it is often the reason. If you add zinc to your dietary intake and your sex life improves, wonderful. If it doesn't, look for another reason, perhaps vitamin E or the unsaturated fatty acids, often known as vitamin F. But don't stop taking your zinc supplement. You still need an adequate amount of zinc in your diet to maintain your good health, sexually as well as otherwise. Ten milligrams three times a day for a total of 30 milligrams daily would be an appropriate amount to take.

A variety of conditions can cause bad breath such as bad teeth, diseased gums, or infected tonsils, but I have found in my practice that a vitamin B shortage is most often to blame. Usually a deficiency of niacin is responsible, but a shortage of vitamin B-6, pyridoxine, can cause bad breath too.

If you do have bad breath, and you have no problems with your teeth, gums or tonsils, then take a high potency B complex such as B-100 or B-50 (Puritan's Pride) with some extra nicotinic acid and pyridoxine three times a day. If your tongue has a fiery red tip or is coated, chances are you need more niacin. If you have a pyridoxine deficiency, you'll probably have swellings of the feet, hands, and around the cheek bones. You'll no doubt have other signs of edema, too. If you're still in doubt, then take an extra supplement of both niacin (in the form of nicotinic acid) and pyridoxine along with your vitamin B complex. You can't take an overdose of any of them. Three hundred milligrams each of nicotinic acid and pyridoxine daily should be sufficient.

* * *

Vitamin C has many functions in the body. It is used in the fundamental metabolic processes of life. It has a special function in the white blood cells of your body to help fight and ward off infection. That may well explain why it is so useful in preventing the common cold. My wife and I both take 3,000 to 6,000 milligrams of vitamin C every day. We always take 3,000 and then up the daily intake to 6,000 at the first sign of any respiratory problem. This stops the oncoming condition cold in its tracks. I frankly cannot recall when either of us has had a cold; it's just been too long ago to remember. Many of my patients could tell you the same thing. If you haven't acquired the vitamin C habit to fight off colds, start right now. Take from 3 to 6 thousand milligrams spread uniformly throughout the day. You'll never regret it.

I cannot explain satisfactorily why vitamin C helps relieve a backache, but I know that it does. Perhaps it is because it helps the body manufacture collagen, a binding substance that helps hold all our cells and bones together. At any rate, if you do have a persistent backache, take vitamin C for it. I guarantee there'll be no dangerous side effects as there are with certain highly advertised over-the-counter non-prescription pills that claim to cure backache for you.

* * *

One of the biggest benefits you could gain from Karen's experience would be to learn how and when to take aspirin. Aspirin does have its valuable uses. It reduces pain, inflammation, and helps to bring down a high fever. But it should not be used in the high dosages as Karen used it.

Nor should you take it when your body is bleeding as hers was. Anyone facing surgery, for instance, should never take aspirin since it could cause severe bleeding during and after the operation. Aspirin can also be life threatening to both the mother and child when it is taken as the time approaches for delivery. Aspirin can cause severe intestinal bleeding which can easily result in anemia.

If you are troubled with painful menstruation, dolomite with its calcium and magnesium content will help you just as it helped Karen. It will also serve as an effective and healthful pain killer in other conditions. So if you're tempted to take a couple of aspirin, reach for half a dozen tablets of dolomite instead. They cannot possibly hurt you. Take enough dolomite tablets to get from 1,000 to 2,000 milligrams of calcium a day. Frankly, I would always prefer the high side myself.

* * *

If you have an infection in the body such as Esther had, vaginal or otherwise, that you have not been able to clear up with any other method, then take a high potency vitamin B supplement such as the B-50 or B-100 three times a day with some dessicated liver and brewer's yeast tablets. They could well be the answer to your problem.

* * *

Since vitamin C is usually the vitamin associated with clearing up infections, you might wonder why Esther's vaginal infection responded to the vitamin B complex the way it did. You might also wonder why a deficiency of the B vitamins caused a vaginal infection in Esther while it caused bad breath and a horrible taste in the mouth for Beulah. And back in Chapter 1, I told you how I got rid of Anna's canker sores by using the vitamin B complex there, too. Let me clear up these points for you right here and now. Such a clarification will help you to better understand the why's and wherefore's of the case histories in the rest of this book.

First of all, let me explain that in infectious diseases, bacteria or viruses will attack the weakest part of the body. The same thing can be said of a food deficiency. It will become evident in that part of the body which is not functioning properly or which is not quite up to par for some reason.

This weakened part of the body usually comes from a deficient nerve and blood supply to the affected area. Now just as long as the person is not deficient in his food intake, or there is no attack by a virus or bacteria, no other condition will show up. Of course, the worst situation will develop when both a food deficiency and a bacterial invasion occur at the same time in the previously weakened area.

Now let's look at these three cases again from this new viewpoint. In Esther's case, the nerve and blood supply to her sex organs was insufficient. Then her dietary intake became deficient in the vitamin B complex, so she developed her vaginal infection.

In Beulah's condition, the nerve and blood supply to her mouth was reduced. Then she became deficient in the vitamin B complex, so her halitosis and the bad taste in her mouth were the result. However, in Anna's case, the insufficient blood and nerve supply followed by the vitamin B complex deficiency gave her canker sores. Why didn't Beulah and Anna develop the same condition in the mouth? Because no two people are alike. No two of us respond in the same way to the same stimuli.

Now it could be that the dietary intake is deficient in some vitamin or mineral first. Then something comes along that lowers the nerve and blood supply to some part of the body. In that situation, the person will usually feel worn out, tired, and generally run down from his deficient food intake. Then when the incident occurs or the situation develops that lowers the nerve and blood supply to some part of the body, a specific ailment will crop up.

That's why my analysis of the dietary intake is important

in my diagnosis and treatment of a patient. It shows which food element is missing from the diet and that's the key to it all. Take the case of Esther's sex organs being predisposed to disease, for instance. An absence of vitamin C rather than the vitamin B complex could just as easily have caused her condition to develop. Since you have no dietary analysis to guide you, you would be wise to take both vitamins B and C if you have any sort of infection.

* * *

Armond's recovery by the use of vitamin C is further evidence of the efficacy of this vitamin to combat infectious conditions. If you have a chronic infection, vitamin C in large quantities can well be the answer to your problem.

* * *

I have used vitamin E successfully for menopausal symptoms in many cases. I normally use from 300 to 1,200 units daily divided into three equal portions for these conditions. I have also found vitamin E beneficial in intermittent claudication, venous thrombosis, and heart trouble. Vitamin E increases the supply of oxygen to the muscles of the body including the heart. It is a natural anticoagulant and helps dissolve blood clots quickly and safely. It improves circulation and is useful in cases of painful leg muscles. I will discuss these conditions along with vitamin E supplementation for them more fully in Chapter 11.

* * *

Just as dolomite was able to help Karen's painful menstruation, so was it able to help the pain and tenderness of Dorothy's cystic mastitis. It is an effective pain killer that is helpful in a great many conditions.

* * *

The value of vitamin E with Gary's poison ivy is only another example of its versatility. It is also valuable to use in cases of sunburn or burns received around the house that do not require a doctor's care. Vitamin E helps heal the skin without leaving any scars.

Laura's case of menstrual problems shows how female complaints can so often be helped by a high potency vitamin B complex taken as a supplement. I have on file case after case of other patients who've been helped the same way. If you suffer from menstrual problems, you could well gain the same benefits for yourself by taking a high potency B complex with dessicated liver and brewer's yeast tablets three times a day.

4

Extraordinary Folk Remedies My Patients Have Told Me About That Worked For Them

As I mentioned previously, I ask all the patients who come to my office if they know of any folk remedy or kitchen medicine that has helped either them or some member of their family. If they do have such a remedy, I get every bit of information about it that I can. I take a complete history of the case, asking the patient not to leave anything out, no matter how trivial or unimportant it might seem to them.

This chapter is a sampling of some of the folk remedies my patients have successfully used themselves. It does not begin to represent all the case histories I have in my files. They would more than fill this book, let alone this chapter. I have done my best to pick the ones I thought would be most helpful to you.

Each case has been authenticated or verified by a witness, usually some other member of the family, although sometimes by me. Verification of the facts is one of the requirements I have always insisted on before I would include a folk remedy and case history in my office files. I should also mention that I have used many of these remedies personally, both on myself and on my patients with excellent results. So now for the first case history...

How Joel treated a wasp sting successfully himself

One Sunday afternoon Joel's grandson, Luke, was bitten on the cheek by a wasp. It hurt like mad and everybody was rushing around trying to figure out what to do for him. I'll let Joel tell you the rest of what happened himself.

"Well, they sprayed his sting with a sunburn spray of some kind, but that didn't help a bit," Joel says. "So they didn't know what to do then. Luckily, I remembered a remedy my mother had used when I got stung on the ankle by a bumblebee once. She covered it with honey to draw out the pain and it disappeared right away.

"I knew there wasn't any use of me suggesting that — what's an old farmer know about medicine, anyway — so I went out to the kitchen and got the honey. I went back into the bedroom where Luke was lying down on the bed crying and I dabbed some honey on the sting before anybody could say anything. Do you know what happened? Why, Luke stopped crying right away.

"Then I made an icebag from a small plastic bag stuffed with ice cubes and held it on his cheek for a while. As soon as his cheek felt good and cold, I dabbed some more honey on the sting. Half an hour later, Luke was up and around playing as if nothing had ever happened."

Greg treats hornet stings with honey, too

Now, whenever a patient tells me about a folk remedy that might benefit some of my other patients, I have the case history — minus the names — mimeographed. Then I place a stack of those mimeographed sheets in the waiting room where people can read them. Luckily Greg's wife, Grace, picked up the case of Joel treating his grandson's wasp sting with honey. Here's why:

A couple of weeks after Grace had been in the office, Greg was mowing their backyard. He was dressed only in a pair of tennis shorts since he was trying to get a good suntan. When his lawnmower bumped a tree, it dislodged a nest of hornets and some of them attacked and stung him.

Now one hornet sting is bad enough, but half a dozen can make even a strong man cry. Greg was in absolute misery. Luckily Grace remembered Joel's case and ran to get some honey. She dabbed honey every place where Greg had been stung. The honey relieved the pain immediately and prevented any swelling. Greg suffered no after effects whatever from the hornet stings.

How my father remarkably cured a bad burn for me

I had almost forgotten this incident until Joel's and Greg's experiences of using honey for wasp and hornet stings. Then it came back to me.

I was born and raised on an Iowa farm. We had no electricity, no indoor plumbing, and no furnace. We used kerosene lamps and carried water from a well. Heat in the winter was supplied by the kitchen range and a potbellied stove in the living room.

My baths in the winter always came on a Saturday night in a small tub behind the potbellied stove. Now my father believed in plenty of heat. He always kept a good fire going in the stoves at all times. This one particular night, that old pot belly stove was cherry red when I got out of my tub. I reached over to pick up my towel, slipped, and lost my balance. As I fell, my right hip hit the cherry red part of the stove. When I jumped away from it, screaming in pain, I left the skin from my hip, about the size of the palm of my hand, on the stove.

This was in December. We lived five miles from town on a dirt road that was snowbound and impassable for a car. There was little to do except suffer the pain. But I could not go to sleep, nor could my parents for I was moaning and groaning in agony. My father had been after my mother to put some honey on the burn to ease the pain, but she thought he was crazy for even suggesting such a thing.

Finally at 3:30 in desperation he went to the kitchen and got the honey despite my mother's objections. He carefully dabbed some over the raw wound and then covered it with a loose bandage. I know it sounds almost unbelievable, but it's true. *The pain ceased immediately.* I fell asleep without any further trouble. The burn healed rapidly without leaving a single scar although it had been at least two inches wide and four inches long.

How Evelyn conquered acne with superb success

As a teenager, Evelyn was bothered with acne all the time. While in her twenties, this problem persisted and hung on in spite of medical treatment and various cosmetic remedies. Her doctor told her that by the time she reached 30, she would surely outgrow her skin problem. But acne continued to trouble Evelyn even into her late thirties.

She had been going to a health food store for her vitamin and mineral supplements. One day she overheard a customer telling the clerk how she'd got over her acne by taking acidophilus capsules.

Evelyn decided to try some herself. To her amazement, after fighting the problem for nearly 30 years, her acne disappeared in less than three weeks. She continues to stay free of it just as long as she takes her acidophilus capsules.

As soon as her teenage daughter began showing signs of acne, Evelyn promptly started her on acidophilus capsules too, with the same happy results. As Evelyn says, the mental and emotional agony — let alone the medical expenses — that a patient goes through with this problem is almost unbelievable. It is her hope, and mine too, that her experience will benefit someone else who is suffering from that same embarrassing problem. That's why her story is in this book.

Opal discovers singular easy-to-use treatment that stops her son's chronic bedwetting

Opal's son, Kevin, had been a chronic bedwetter for years. She tried almost everything, but to no avail. She had taken him to several doctors, but had been unable to receive any help for him.

Then a craze started at Kevin's school. The children would buy cinnamon oil, soak toothpicks in it, and chew on them. Kevin seemed to have an insatiable craving for cinnamon, Opal said. He would raid her spice cabinet for it and sprinkle ground cinnamon on his hand and lick it. He would also chew on pieces of cinnamon bark that Opal kept in her spice jar.

Shortly after this cinnamon fad started, Kevin stopped

wetting his bed. This remedy seemed almost too simple to be true, so they tested it by stopping his consumption of the cinnamon bark for a few days. Sure enough, he started wetting the bed again. As soon as he started chewing on the cinnamon bark once more, he stopped.

When Opal told me about this, I mimeographed Kevin's case history and placed it in the waiting room as usual. One of my patients had an eight-year-old girl with the same problem. After reading about Kevin's case, she went straight to the health food store from my office and bought some cinnamon bark for her daughter to chew on. In only a few nights she stopped wetting the bed, too.

How Willa amazingly rid herself of her ugly warts

Willa had been troubled for more than four years with warts on her left hand. There were more than a dozen in number, large, troublesome, and ugly. Willa often bumped them while she was working, sometimes causing them to crack open and bleed.

She had tried various remedies such as garlic oil, castor oil, vitamin E ointment, fish liver oil with vitamin A for her warts, but none of these seemed to work for her. She went to a dermatologist but without success there either.

Then she heard about a person who'd gotten rid of warts in short order by eating four or five tablespoons of asparagus twice a day. Willa decided it was worth a try. She made a sort of puree out of some frozen asparagus in her blender. It took two months but the warts disappeared. When she started her asparagus treatment, she had 15 large warts on her hand with a number of small ones that appeared to be getting bigger.

I looked at her hand myself the other day and all that she had left were some little white spots like freckle marks. I could not find one wart and I could well remember what her hand had looked like before.

Muscular pain swiftly surrenders to new kind of tea

A few weeks ago, Maude's right arm received a bad sprain in an automobile accident. A few days later, she developed a severe muscle pain just below the shoulder in her back. She figured she must have pulled a muscle since it felt like a bad ankle or wrist sprain. It hurt in every position making it extremely difficult for her to sleep at night. Her doctor told her that she had a muscle strain and recommended massage and a muscular ointment. This did not seem to help at all.

Then a friend heard of Maude's predicament and brought her over some comfrey tea. She told Maude how it had helped her muscular aches and pains and asked her to try it. Although Maude was skeptical of the medicinal qualities of comfrey tea, she agreed to drink several cups of it throughout the day. Toward evening the pain had begun to ease and she was able to sleep quite comfortably that night for the first time since her accident. By morning the pain was nearly gone.

On the second day Maude drank three cups of the comfrey tea, morning, noon, and night, instead of coffee. The pain continued to lessen. She kept up the treatment and within the week the muscle was healed and the pain was completely gone.

Dave's new method resolves bladder infection

Dave had been troubled with a chronic bladder infection for more than 30 years. He had taken medicine for it continually which did help to keep the condition under control, but never healed it.

Then he read in a health magazine that fresh cranberries were good for chronic bladder infections, so he decided to try them. He bought a couple of small bags of cranberries, crushed them, and mixed them with enough raw honey to make them palatable. He ate a dish of them every day for a week and his bladder infection ceased to exist.

When that happened, Dave went all out and bought a case of cranberries at the store. He ground them in his food blender and mixed them with raw honey. Then he put the mixture up in cartons and stored them in his freezer.

Now at the first sign of any possible trouble, he eats a dish of the cranberry and honey mixture. He sometimes mixes it with plain yogurt for he says it makes a very satisfying bedtime snack.

The last seige Dave had of bladder infection has been

more than a year ago and he was able to clear it up in less than twelve hours with the cranberry and honey mixture. He has not taken any medication in that time. Dave no longer eats the cranberry and honey mixture every day; instead, he watches his urine carefully. At the first sign of a change in its odor, he eats a dish of his cranberry and honey mixture and the infection never develops.

A mother's unusually safe and easy-to-use remedy for her children's diarrhea

Diarrhea can be a most troublesome problem, especially for young school children. Penny told me that every time she turned around, it seemed as if her two youngsters were coming home from school suffering from diarrhea. Various medicines gave no relief and did nothing but upset their stomachs.

Then a friend of hers ("I used to call her a health food freak until this happened," Penny says) told her to try feeding her children yogurt for their diarrhea. "And lo and behold, it worked," Penny says. "Now when they have trouble I feed them yogurt for breakfast, lunch and dinner. So far, only one day's treatment is all it takes. I often use the kinds with fruit in them since the children like them much better. They work, too."

Patient swears by unique arthritis treatment

Pete has been bothered off and on with rheumatism and arthritis in his back for a number of years. A few months ago it got so bad he could hardly get in and out of his car.

Pete has always liked to bowl and is in several leagues, so he bowls two and three times a week. This time his problem became so serious that he was afraid he would have to give up his bowling. His wife and family tried to get him to come to me, but although they are all patients of mine, Pete himself has never been "sold" on chiropractic, so he said he'd figure out something for himself.

Then one of the fellows on his team told Pete how he had been able to control his own arthritis by drinking alfalfa tea.

Pete not only tried the alfalfa tea, but he also ate alfalfa seeds for his arthritis, too. He would grind up three or four table-spoons of them every day and eat them with yogurt or fruit or mix them with milk.

The use of alfalfa worked wonderfully for Pete. His back is in excellent shape again. He did not have to give up his bowling and he's still knocking the pins down in his leagues. Pete is only a young 68 years old, too.

Eighty-two-year old woman gets rid of nausea and dizziness by unusually easy-to-use methods

Nell is 82 years old. During the past several years, her ten-dency toward morning nausea was getting worse. She also suffered from some dizziness. She had had one slight stroke al-ready. Nell did a lot of reading of health magazines and read one article that recommended using the entire peel of lemons and oranges by grating them into the juice. The article said the rind of citrus fruit was good for nausea and dizziness.

Nell decided to try the remedy. She grates the rind of one lemon or an orange into her fruit salad or mixed fruit cup each day. She also chews and sucks on the rind of an orange. She says this has cleared up her nausea and dizziness completely.

Kidney problems resolved by unusual home remedy

I have had several people tell me their experiences about clearing up kidney problems with kidney bean water. The first to do so was Iris.

Iris had been bothered by a dull ache across the small of her back and pain and tenderness over the kidney region for six or seven months. Her urine was cloudy, had a bad odor, and burned whenever she went to the bathroom.

She read in a health magazine about using kidney bean pods to clear up the urine and clean out the kidneys. She wanted to try it, so she planted some kidney beans along in the latter part of May. During the month of August she was able to get six pickings of the ripe kidney beans.

To make the kidney bean water, Iris used half a dozen bean pods to a quart of water. She boiled this for several hours, strained it, and let it stand for at least two hours until it was cool. Then she drank a glass of the kidney bean water every two hours.

After a few glasses of the kidney bean water, her urine, which had previously been cloudy with a foul smell, became crystal clear and had no bad odor at all. Iris continued this treatment for a week and her kidney problem and backache cleared up completely. She has had no more trouble with her kidneys since then.

Harry developed a kidney infection about a month before the kidney bean pods would be ready in his garden. His doctor treated him with antibiotics, but the infection did not clear up.

As soon as the kidney bean pods were ripe, Harry made some of the kidney bean water, just as Iris had done, and drank a quart of it every day for two weeks.

At the end of that time, he returned to his doctor for a check-up, and found his kidneys to be completely free of infection, even though he had not taken his antibiotics for close to a month. His doctor was quite pleased with the results. Harry said he never told him about drinking the kidney bean water.

Phenomenal treatment heals spider bite

Last summer while on a picnic on Sunday afternoon with his family, Art was bitten by a black widow spider. By the time they got back home, his leg was badly swollen in the area of the bite. It' was already festering and had red lines shooting out from it. Art was sweating profusely and was short of breath.

Since it was a Sunday, Art didn't even try to call a doctor. Instead, he took massive doses of liquid vitamin C by the tablespoonful every ten or fifteen minutes for the first two hours and then every hour after that.

His wife, Rhoda, also mixed some rose hip powder (which contains vitamin C) with some cold cream and applied it to the bite. By that evening Art was feeling much better. By the next morning he had completely recovered.

Fay's troublesome B O problem remarkably solved by rare mineral

Fay had always been troubled with excessive body odor for as long as she could remember. She bathed regularly each day and was meticulous about her personal hygiene. She had tried a variety of deodorants, but none of them seemed strong enough to overcome her own body odor. Fay was in a vicious cycle: the more she worried about her problem, the more she perspired, and the worse her problem became.

One day Fay read a small article in a health magazine about a young man who'd had the same problem. This fellow had been troubled with excessive underarm perspiration and body odor along with perspiring feet and a bad foot odor. He had used various dusting powders and well-known deodorants, many of which had given him a bad skin rash, with no success at all. Then he started taking 30 milligrams of zinc daily for another problem. In a few weeks his body odor subsided and went away completely.

Fay decided to try the zinc therapy herself. She also took 30 milligrams a day and at the end of only two weeks, she had no more offensive body odor either. She could undress at night after a hard day's work washing and ironing, cooking and cleaning house to find that her armpits smelled as fresh as if she'd just bathed. Her undergarments smelled clean, too, as if they'd just been washed.

Benefits You Can Gain from the Case Histories in This Chapter

Honey is useful to take the pain out of stings and burns that are not bad enough to need a doctor's attention. It is certainly an inexpensive remedy to use. A couple of my patients tell me they have used molasses with the same good results. This could well be, but personally I still prefer the honey.

* * *

When I first heard of the cinnamon bark treatment for bedwetting, I was quite dubious as usual about the efficacy of this folk remedy. Since then, I have received reports from several other patients whose children were bothered the same way. They tell me they have all received good results from this folk remedy. In most cases, their children stopped wetting the bed altogether. In others, the cinnamon reduced the frequency until it would happen only once in a while. If you have children with this problem, you can try cinnamon bark too. It could easily be the solution to this problem and end your child's misery and embarrassment.

* * *

I've heard of all sorts of remedies for warts over the years — garlic oil, castor oil, vitamin E oil, and fish liver oil with vitamin A, that often do work for some people. However, if you've been unsuccessful with all of these, try the asparagus treatment for yourself. It surely can't hurt you, and that's for sure.

* * *

Comfrey tea, a natural herbal tea, is a marvelous alternative to aspirin or pain pills. It is quite palatable and even children accept it. This is once when you can offer a child tea without worrying about its bad effects as you have to do with regular tea or coffee. Add a teaspoon of honey to each cup of tea in stead of sugar. Honey is also noted as a soothing remedy for muscular aches and pains.

* * *

Cranberries are useful in combatting any infection in the body because they help acidify the body and make the urine acid. Sickness and infection always occur in the body with an alkaline urine.

For instance, when a common cold is on the way, the urine reaction will change from acid to alkaline, and will continue to be alkaline for several days in advance of the appearance of the cold. During recovery from the cold, the urine will shift from an alkaline reaction to an acid one. If cranberries aren't for you, then you can drink grape juice, apple juice, or a teaspoon of apple cider vinegar in a glass of water. These help to acidify the body fluids and the urine too to help fight off infections.

Yogurt can be valuable for a variety of intestinal problems other than diarrhea, too. For instance, infections caused by the fungus monilia albicans often result from the use of oral antibiotics. The fungus multiplies rapidly in the large intestines and causes severe itching around the anus. It is easily transmitted by the fingers and fingernails and can result in an irritating vaginal infection. The consumption of yogurt or acidophilus capsules restores the proper intestinal flora in which the fungus monilia albicans cannot live.

* * *

I have run into a variety of folk remedies for arthritis over the years. Some seem to work better for some people, while other remedies work better for others. It all depends on what food factor is missing from the diet.

I have used alfalfa tablets successfully for rheumatism and arthritis in some cases. Alfalfa is rich in natural vitamins and minerals. It is often used as the base for multi-vitamin tablets by several leading vitamin manufacturing companies.

* * *

Vitamin P, or the bioflavonoids, is the element found in citrus rinds that was so helpful to Nell in combatting her nausea and dizziness. I have found the same treatment to be useful in treating morning sickness in pregnant women.

The bioflavonoids can also be taken in a tablet form. If you take a vitamin C preparation made from natural sources such as rose hips, for example, some bioflavonoids will be included. The synthetic vitamin C, ascorbic acid, does not contain them. However, patients of mine tell me they get better results when they use the lemon or orange rind instead of the tablet for their spells of nausea, dizziness and morning sickness.

* * *

I have had quite a few patients tell me about their experiences drinking kidney bean water. One woman was able to clear up the swelling in her feet and ankles in about two and one half weeks by drinking it. Others tell me that cloudy, bad smelling urine will clear up and become clean and crystal clear.

Everyone says the kidney bean pods must be fresh. This

folk remedy might be a bit inconvenient for you to use, but if you have kidney problems that haven't been resolved by anything else, a couple of rows of kidney beans in your backyard or even in the back porch flower box might be well worth that extra effort it takes.

* * *

Vitamin C is one of the most effective healing agents that can be used to combat infections and poisons. Doctor Fred Klenner, a North Carolina medical doctor, is a pioneer in the use of vitamin C to combat a variety of illnesses. He has used it to heal a man who had been bitten by an extremely poisonous puss caterpillar. Dr. Klenner injected 12,000 milligrams of ascorbic acid into the bloodstream to neutralize the poison.

"Except for the vitamin C, this man would have died from shock and asphyxiation," Dr. Klenner says.

In another case, a four-year-old girl was bitten on the leg by a poisonous snake. When she was brought to Dr. Klenner's office, she was vomiting and crying with pain and fright. While Dr. Klenner waited for an antivenom skin test reaction to determin which antivenom to use, he gave her an injection of 4,000 milligrams of vitamin C. Even before the antivenom was given to her, the child had stopped crying and vomiting. She was laughing and drinking a glass of orange juice. A second injection of vitamin C restored her to normal.

An economical way to have plenty of vitamin C on hand for an emergency is to buy it in a powder form from the health food store. A tablespoon of the powder can be spooned into a glass of water to be taken as often as necessary. Vitamin C has also been found to speed up the healing of burns when it is taken orally.

* * *

Although I've used zinc for other problems, some of which I've already told you about, I have never had a patient come to me primarily for the problem of foot odor or body odor. If you have either one of these, take 30 milligrams of zinc each day for 30 days and judge the results for yourself, just as Fay did. You could be pleasantly surprised too, just as she was. But don't expect the zinc to take away the natural, normal body odors. It won't do that.

5

How to Treat Colds, Hay Fever, Allergies and Sinus Problems with Marked Success

People who suffer from hay fever will tell you there is no disease more dreadful known to man. Those who are plagued with chronic colds, allergies, sinusitis, and the like also know that such ailments can be extremely irritating. People who have never suffered with such problems as these have no concept of the misery a person can go through. As one of my patients who used to have hay fever told me, "The trouble with hay fever is you never look sick enough to get any sympathy or understanding, but you never feel well enough to do anything either."

If you do suffer with one of these respiratory ailments, I heartily recommend that you use one of the appropriate remedies given in this chapter. It may well be the solution to the problem you've put up with for so long.

How Quincy incredibly avoids Winter colds

A little more than ten years ago, Quincy was stricken with a bad case of the flu. His doctor placed him in the hospital and gave him shots for it. The side effect of his medication was an intestinal dysentery that left Quincy in an extremely weakened condition. After he left the hospital, he spent another two weeks at home recuperating. During that time he developed a chronic cold that he couldn't get rid of no matter what he did.

Even after he'd gone back to work at the post office, Quincy felt weak and run down; he still had his cold. One day his supervisor, a patient of mine, recommended to Quincy that he come see me. He told Quincy he'd been coming to me for more than three years and he'd not had even the faintest sign of a cold or any other respiratory ailment in that time. So Quincy called to ask for an appointment.

My physical examination revealed that Quincy was still in a weakened condition and that he had not completely recovered from his previous illness. Dietary analysis showed him to be deficient in all his vitamins and minerals, but especially so in his intake of vitamin C.

I supplemented Quincy's diet with a high potency supplement of all the vitamins and minerals to build up his health and help him regain his strength. For his cold I specifically gave him 6,000 milligrams — 1,500 milligrams four times a day — of vitamin C for the first three months. Then I lowered his intake to 3,000 milligrams a day, which he has been taking ever since.

Now let's look at the results. First of all, Quincy gained back his pep, his energy, his go-power, and he felt like a new person at the end of only 30 days. He has not had any sign of a serious cold since he started on his high intake of vitamin C each day, and that was nearly ten years ago.

If he ever does have even the faintest sign of the sniffles, Quincy ups his vitamin C to at least 8,000 milligrams a day by taking 500 milligrams every waking hour. His sniffles will disappear withi 24 hours and a cold never develops. He puts in eight hours a day and has not missed a day's work with a respiratory ailment since he began doctoring with me. He is much more active and healthy than a lot of men I know who are in their early sixties, as Quincy is.

Druggist's sore throat amazingly vanishes in one day with new method

Although Tom is not a patient of mine, we go to the same church, play golf together, and enjoy each other's company. Actually, his views of sickness and health are diametrically opposed to mine since he is a pharmacist.

I saw Tom one Sunday at church and he was chewing up cough drops by the handful. He'd had a sore throat for a week, he said, and nothing he'd taken had been able to shake it. "Tom, why don't you take some vitamin C instead of all those cough drops?" I asked. "You'd probably get rid of your sore throat overnight."

The next Sunday I saw Tom again. He had no sign of his sore throat. When I asked him about it, he grinned sheepishly and said, "Well, I sure hate to tell you this, Jim, but your vitamin C got rid of it for me."

"I went down to the store Monday morning, still thinking about what you'd said. I grabbed a bottle of vitamin C on the way through the store to my office. I took two 250 milligram tablets, crushed them in a glass of water, and made a solution to gargle with. After I did that I took one 250 milligram tablet orally. My throat felt better within the hour. I continued to gargle with vitamin C solution and took a tablet every hour throughout the day. By quitting time my sore throat was completely gone.

"I now keep a bottle of vitamin C on my desk. At the first sign of a tickle in my throat I reach for a vitamin C tablet instead of a cough drop as I used to."

John's sinus problem solved with amazing results after years of misery

When John finally came to see me, he had been suffering from a chronic sinus ailment for many years. In fact, his condition was so bad ulcers had developed in his nasal passages. Much of the septum between the right and left nasal cavities had been destroyed. Drainage from his sinuses was constant in the winter months. This drainage would infect the bronchial tubes in the upper part of his lungs. He had had pneumonia twice as a result.

Initially, treatment had consisted of sulfa, both orally and as an ointment for John's nasal passages, but this gave him only temporary relief. He then moved to New Mexico, hoping the dry arid climate would help his condition, but there was still no improvement. His doctors in Santa Fe treated him with penicillin, terramycin, aureomycin, streptomycin and a variety of other drugs, but again he received only temporary benefits.

By this time John decided he was no better off in the west

than he'd been in Missouri, so he returned to his beloved Ozarks. Then, upon the recommendation of a friend, he came to my office. I found that John was extremely low in vitamin A. I started him off with 10,000 units a day, twice the recommended daily allowance, for a month, but we saw very little improvement. I slowly increased his daily intake up to 60,000 units which is 12 times the government's minimum daily requirement. Then his sinus condition began to improve.

John has been under my care for a little more than one year now. He has had no more trouble with his condition since we started using vitamin A in such large quantities. His sinus drainage has ceased and the nasal ulcers have all healed. Of course, the perforations in the septum still exist, but that is to be expected. I now have dropped his daily intake of vitamin A down to 25,000 units, which is still five times the minimum daily requirement, but I do not foresee going any lower than that, at least not for a long time.

John's case was slow to respond until I increased his vitamin A intake up to 60,000 units a day. His condition improved steadily from then on. You might think a year is too long to get well, but please remember what I said previously: it takes about one month of treatment for every year the patient has had the condition.

Two novel approaches to sinus problems

A high potency vitamin A supplement is the best solution for chronic sinusitis since it is necessary for the restoration of the mucous membranes. However, two of my patients told me about their solutions to their sinus problems, so I want to pass them along for your benefit. You could use them in addition to taking vitamin A.

Kathleen tells me she has found orange peelings to be the best remedy she has ever used for her sinuses. She keeps the peelings in her refrigerator until she has enough to work with. Then she cuts them in little pieces and soaks them in apple cider vinegar for several hours. After that, they go into a pan of raw honey and she cooks them down slowly, not quite to the candy stage. She keeps these in her refrigerator and eats them as necessary to control her sinuses. She says they keep her nasal passages clean and clear and allow her to sleep without stopping up at night.

Peggy uses garlic for her sinus problems. She read that garlic pills were good for colds and sinus infections, so she decided to try them. She says they work fine for her. She takes eight capsules a day, two with each meal and two before going to bed. They keep her sinuses clear and stop the drainage, which is usually so much worse at night. As long as she takes the garlic, her sinuses do not bother her. The moment she stops taking it, her sinuses fill up again, causing her to have headaches and nasal congestion.

Several cases of hay fever whipped by uncommon treatment

As I said previously, hay fever is one of the most dreadful diseases known to man. People who suffer from this ailment hate to see the hay fever season approach, for they well remember the swollen watery eyes and the stuffy congested nose from past experience. Let me tell you about the results I've obtained in just a few of the many cases of hay fever I've been able to help. If you suffer from hay fever yourself, one of them could well be the answer for you.

1. *Hay fever cleared up with vitamins A and E.* At the age of 30, Maxine suddenly came down with hay fever for the first time. She had all the symptoms: swollen watery eyes, sneezing, and congested nose. She was absolutely miserable. Her doctor tried hay fever shots and various pills, but nothing helped her. By the middle of October her hay fever let up, but she dreaded the thought of the next summer, the hay fever season, and more of the same.

A friend suggested to her that she might be suffering from a nutritional deficiency that caused her allergy, so Maxine came to see me. I found her to be deficient in both vitamins A and E. I started her off on 20,000 units of vitamin A and 400 units of vitamin E divided up into four equal amounts each day. I gradually built these up until she was taking 50,000 units of A and 1,200 units of E daily about a month before the hay fever season began.

Maxine had some of her symptoms of hay fever that summer but they were much milder than before. She continued taking her vitamin A and E supplements throughout the winter. The second summer she came through the hay fever season with no trouble at all.

Maxine also gained some valuable fringe benefits from her vitamin supplements. Her eyes, which had bothered her since childhood, are now completely normal. They are no longer sensitive to light, nor do they tear excessively as before. Her skin previously had been dry and her hair coarse. Now her complexion is moist and smooth without any creams and lotions. Her blackheads and pimples have all disappeared, too. Maxine's hair no longer needs additional oils. It now has a natural sheen all its own. She no longer keeps it cut short as she did for so many years. Since it is now so thick and luxuriant, she lets her hair grow long which greatly pleases her husband.

2. *Vitamin C works to cure Tony's allergy.* For years Tony suffered from hay fever and various other allergies. From August to the end of September was the hardest time of all. He would be in misery because of ragweed. He could hardly breathe...his eyes would be red and swollen...he had terrible headaches from the congestion in his sinuses. Tony often had to stay home from work taking all sorts of pills to try to help his condition. None of them ever worked for him.

When his boss told him he would have to let him go unless he could be on the job every day, Tony went to see an allergy specialist. The various tests showed he was allergic to almost everything: trees, plants, grass, ragweed, mold, mildew, even dust.

Tony started taking shots for his condition and in the beginning he had good results from his treatment. The first summer he took the shots he had very little reaction to the ragweed when it came.

However, the next summer the allergy was back just as bad as it had been in the beginning in spite of the shots. Evidently his body had become immune to the serum, but not to the ragweed.

The next March Tony came to me for help. He had read an

article stating that many allergies have a nutritional basis. Dietary analysis of his food intake showed him to be extremely deficient in vitamin C. I started Tony on 4,000 milligrams of vitamin C along with the bioflavonoids. I built this up to 8,000 milligrams a day by June. He went through the entire hay fever season this last summer and fall and sneezed only a few times, and he did not miss one single day of work.

3. *Two other cases of hay fever solved by vitamin supplements.* Joy had been bothered by hay fever for more than ten years. I gave her additional vitamin C right while she was suffering from an acute attack. Her recovery was almost instantaneous. Within a few hours after taking her first vitamin C supplement, she could breathe through her nose. Her eyes stopped itching and she got a good night's sleep for the first time in weeks.

The second case is that of a 70-year-old woman, Ina, who'd had hay fever every summer and fall for as long as she could remember. Although she lived on a farm, she could not do any outside work at all during the hay fever season. She did not dare go near the haymow. The presence of a cat would make her sneeze incessantly, and her eyes would water and swell so that she could hardly see.

Ina was deficient in both vitamins A and C. I gave her additional amounts of each and she is no longer troubled by her allergy after all these years. Hay, cats, goldenrod, ragweed, or other air impurities no longer bother her. She has not had a cold since she started taking her vitamins.

4. *Hay Fever gives in to honey and honey comb.* In cases of hay fever where I can find no major vitamin deficiency, I have discovered that raw honey, honey cappings, or honey comb will work extremely well to prevent or relieve hay fever symptoms.

You may recall that I told you in Chapter 2 how Vince and his son got rid of their hay fever by taking two tablespoons of raw honey each day. I first got this remedy from a patient. After seeing the results Vince and his son got, I decided to investigate the use of honey to prevent hay fever and other allergies even further.

I have talked to more than two dozen beekeepers in Iowa, Missouri, and Florida. Not a single one of them has ever been troubled with hay fever, or any other allergy for that matter. Not only that, they all seem to be remarkably free from colds. Of course, they all eat honey and chew on honey comb and honey cappings.

In 1965, I developed a mild nasal congestion that bothered me every spring and fall for several years. Each year it got a little worse, and since I was already taking a full supplement of vitamins and minerals, I turned to honey for the remedy. I soon found it worked like a charm for me, too.

Now I use honey all the time instead of sugar. I use it in my tea and on cereals, too. My wife uses it in place of sugar in all her cooking and baking. I also chew honey comb or honey cappings three times a day during the hay fever season or whenever I get the slightest hint of nasal congestion. It has worked wonderfully for me as well as for my other patients who've used it.

Asthma patient quickly helped by singular treatment

Vicki had been bothered with asthma since she was two years old. When her parents brought her to me in despair, she was 20 pounds underweight. The slightest exertion would bring on a wheezing attack. Vicki had been on medication for years, but no permanent relief had ever been obtained. Her face was drawn and pale. She had a hearing problem and was a grade behind in school because of missing so many classes. More than once her parents had rushed her to the hospital for emergency injections of adrenalin during an acute asthmatic attack.

Vick's dietary habits were terrible. She hated fresh fruit and vegetables. Her parents felt sorry for her, so they gave in to her wishes all the time. As a result, Vicki was literally living on a diet of man-made carbohydrates — foods that were loaded down with refined white sugar.

I found her to be in need of additional vitamins A, C, E, and the B complex. She was also highly deficient in calcium and magnesium. Her sugar intake was far too high.

I asked Vicki's parents to eliminate all refined white sugar and products containing it from her diet at once. I also asked them to make sure she got plenty of fresh fruit and vegetables. I gave her 6,000 milligrams of vitamin C, 20,000 units of vitamin A, 300 units of E, and a high potency vitamin B complex as well as some dessicated liver and yeast tablets on a daily basis. Her calcium and magnesium deficiency was corrected by dolomite.

In less than three months, Vicki had stopped wheezing and suffered no more asthma attacks, even after running and playing with the other children at recess time and after school. The color came back to her cheeks where before they'd been pale and lifeless — the color of chalk.

At the end of nine months of treatment, Vicki was up to the normal weight for her height and age. One year after she first came to my office, she was a normal healthy child who bore absolutely no resemblance to the skinny, underweight, asthmatic child who'd first come to see me. She never once during that year had to have one adrenalin shot. Nor has she had to have one since then, either.

How Everett's shortness of breath was relieved in extremely short order

Everett, too, was an asthmatic. He had been troubled with it for years, but had done nothing for it except to use mists and sprays to try and keep the bronchial passages clear. He came to me for a cardiovascular problem rather than asthma. His main complaint about his asthma was shortness of breath.

Everett was extremely deficient in vitamin E so I placed him on 400 units a day for the first month, 800 for the second, and 1,200 units a day for the third month of treatment. As soon as we went to 1,200 units a day, Everett noticed his asthma was much better and he could breathe more easily.

Then he decided to experiment on his own — which I do not advise anyone with a cardiovascular condition to do. He reasoned that if 1,200 units a day would help his asthmatic problem, then more of it would be helpful in case of an acute asthmatic attack. So he did just that. He took 2,400 units during an asthmatic seizure. Within half an hour his attack was over and he suffered no side effects whatever. He has done this successfully on several occasions since then. His asthmatic attacks have also diminished in both number and severity since he has been taking vitamin E.

I certainly do not recommend such high consumption of vitamin E unless you are under a doctor's supervision if you have a history of high blood pressure or rheumatic heart disease. If you have either one of these, then vitamin E could cause some problems for you, as I mention in Chapter 9 on page 134.

How You Can Benefit from the Case Histories in This Chapter

Vitamin C is the most effective "medicine" you can take for a cold. To avoid a cold, take at least 3,000 milligrams a day — 1,000 each for breakfast, dinner, and supper — all the time. Then if you do develop signs of a cold, take another 500 to 1,000 milligrams each hour until the symptoms disappear. Don't give up too soon. Sometimes the virus is a little stubborn, but vitamin C always wins out just as long as you don't stop taking it too soon.

If you have a sore throat, you also can use a vitamin C solution to gargle just as Tom did besides taking vitamin C, just as you would for a cold. Crush two tablets of uncoated vitamin C in a glass of water and stir vigorously. Or you can use two teaspoons of vitamin C powder to a glass. This beats any commercial gargle you can buy. It's a lot cheaper and much more effective.

Above all, don't let your doctor give you a shot of penicillin or some other antibiotic for a cold. Antibiotics do nothing for your cold since they act only against bacteria, and colds are caused by viruses. You can only be hurt, not only from the possible side effects, but also because recent scientific tests show that people who take antibiotics for the common cold take more time to recover than people who don't. Not only that, your pocketbook will suffer too. Vitamin C is safer, cheaper, and more effective for your cold than any shot can ever be.

Vitamin A is the best treatment I know of to heal irritated mucous membranes, no matter where they are. It promotes healthy functioning of the mucous membranes of the nasal cavities, eyes, ears, sinuses, the respiratory and urinary tracts. A deficiency of vitamin A will cause inflammation and infection, especially of the ear and nasal cavities.

As an adult, you need not be concerned about taking too much vitamin A unless you take at least 100,000 units a day for *many, many* months, according to the 12th edition of *The Merck Manual**, which is known in the medical profession as the "Physician's Prescription Bible."

Early clinical symptoms of taking 100,000 units of vitamin A for *many, many* months could be sparse coarse hair, loss of hair in the eyebrows, a rough dry skin, and cracked lips. However, to set your mind at ease on this subject, let me tell you that in all the history of medicine there are only about 24 recorded cases of persons who took too much vitamin A and suffered any distress. No fatalities have ever been reported. Signs and symptoms of vitamin A overdosage disappeared within one to four weeks after stopping the consumption of vitamin A.

As long as you keep your vitamin A intake below that level, you will have no problem. You need to concern yourself more with not getting enough vitamin A in your diet. Here's why:

Studies conducted in Canada show a high percentage of Canadians did not have enough vitamin A in their bodies at the time of death. Dr. T. Keith Murray, Chief of the Nutritional Research Division of the Canadian Food and Drug Directorate in Ottawa, says there is a tremendous incidence of vitamin A deficiency in Canadians. He also says in effect that the same condition is no doubt prevalent in the United States.

Dr. Murray suspects that environmental pollution, drugs, pesticides, and food additives to prevent spoilage are to blame. He thinks these additives have cut down on our ability to use the vitamin A we consume efficiently, or in some cases, that we might be burning it up too fast in our bodies.

---

*Merck, Sharp & Dohme Research Laboratories, Rahway, New Jersey, a Division of Merck & Company, Inc., 1972.

Professor Jean Mayer says insufficient vitamin A is one of the main causes of blindness in Americans today. Vitamin A is one of two main vitamins most Americans do not get enough of; vitamin C is the other.

* * *

As you can see from the way these different cases of hay fever were relieved, treatment all depends upon the patient's dietary deficiency. In some instances, vitamins A and E solved the problem; in others, vitamin C did the work, while in still others a combination of A and C was necessary. If you have hay fever, then it would be wise for you to take the shotgun approach and use large amounts of all these vitamins: A, C, and E. You might consider taking at least 30,000 units of A, 3 to 5,000 milligrams of C, and 800 to 1,200 units of E as a general guideline to go by.

If I had hay fever, I would also definitely consider the use of honey, honey cappings and honey comb. Honey is a natural food and so much better for you than sugar that there is really no valid comparison of the two. Again I say, whatever you do, don't give up too soon. If you do, you'll always have your hay fever to contend with.

Although asthma, just like hay fever, is an allergy, I have found so often that a patient can overcome that allergy when he follows these four simple rules:

1. *Eats the proper food, especially fresh fruits and fresh vegetables.*

2. *Gets the proper vitamins and minerals in his diet.* A, C, E, sometimes the B complex as in Vicki's case, calcium and magnesium seem to be the ones most often needed. Vitamins A and C help to desensitize the body and reduce the allergic manifestations. Vitamins C and E, especially E, also increase the oxygen supply to the body. That is why the large doses of vitamin E helped to relieve Everett's asthmatic attacks.

3. *Eliminates refined white sugar and all products containing it from the diet.* Honey can be used as a natural sweetener. It is valuable in treating asthma just as in treating hay fever.

4. *Avoids packaged and processed man-made foods as much as possible.* A good rule of thumb to follow is *eat food that is born — not made.*

Searching for a specific allergen in the diet or the environment can be expensive, time-consuming, frustrating, and often painful. I've had patients who've had dozens of skin tests without ever discovering the specific allergen that was causing their problem. These tests are both painful and expensive. I've also had patients who thought they could not eat eggs, bread, cheese, milk, and so on, yet who found they could when they followed the four simple rules I've just listed. In most cases I have handled, the patient's asthma has been completely relieved or the severity of the condition greatly reduced by these simple measures.

❅ ❅ ❅

I want to say a bit more here about refined white sugar. I have found that colds, tonsillitis, sinus infections, various respiratory allergies, asthma, and other bronchial conditions with mucous discharges are always much worse in people who are heavy users of white refined sugar. When a person gives up sugar altogether and uses honey instead, these conditions can be cured much more easily and rapidly.

I have had many patients recover quickly from such allergies as asthma, bronchitis, hay fever, eczema, hives, and migraine or nervous headaches when they eliminate all refined white sugar and food products containing sugar from their diets.

6

How to Rid Yourself
of Upper Digestive Tract Problems
Permanently with Fantastic Results

I have never kept track of what percentage of my practice is devoted to digestive disorders, but I know that a great many of my patients do come to me with gastro-intestinal problems.

I've had patients who've used anti-acids for ten to twenty years to relieve heartburn, but they still had it when they came to me. Why? Others come with a history of using laxatives all their life, yet they still suffer from constipation. How come? In both cases, for the simple reason that drugs for ailments of the digestive tract treat only the symptoms. They give only temporary relief to the patient. Drugs do not offer a person any lasting benefits because they never eliminate the cause of the problem.

In this chapter and the next, I will cover the most common ailments of the upper and lower digestive tracts I've treated in my practice. You'll see from the case histories that you do not have to suffer with canker sores, bleeding gums, heartburn, indigestion, constipation, diarrhea, and so on. You'll also find that you need not turn to drugs to obtain relief. And you'll also discover that almost every single digestive ailment is caused by not eating enough of the right kinds of food, including vitamins and minerals, or by eating too much of the wrong kinds of food.

How I got fabulous results with canker sores: four case histories

Martin came to see me for high blood pressure. While taking his case history, I found he was allergic to tomatoes. Although he liked them very much, he said he had given up eating them altogether since they caused him to have such extremely painful canker sores.

I told Martin he did not necessarily have to give up tomatoes, for I had found that the bacteria in yogurt, known as lactobacillus acidophilus, would heal canker sores and they would probably also prevent them. I suggested to Martin that he eat some yogurt each day and experiment for himself to find out. He did so and found to his great joy that as long as he ate yogurt, he could also eat tomatoes. However, if he tried eating tomatoes again without yogurt, he would always break out with canker sores.

Ruth brought her 11-year-old son, Allen, to me to see if I could do something for his canker sores. Repeated trips to doctors and dentists had failed to reveal the cause of his problem or any possible remedy. Allen was troubled with canker sores all the time, week after week, month after month. His mother suspected a food allergy, but she had been unable to tie his condition to any specific food that might be causing it.

I told Ruth and Allen about Martin's case and how he was able to prevent canker sores by eating yogurt. Although Allen's canker sores did not seem to be caused by a food allergy as Martin's was, he and his mother decided to try the yogurt therapy.

Allen's relief from canker sores was almost instantaneous. In only three days they were gone completely. As long as he eats a little every day, he does not suffer with his former canker sores.

Irvin had the same problem Martin and Allen had. His canker sores could not be traced to any specific food. However, when I suggested yogurt to Irvin, he turned up his nose in disgust. He didn't even like the sound of the name.

But I was still able to offer a solution for Irvin, just as I had for Martin and Allen. Since the active ingredient in yogurt is the lactobacillus acidophilus, Irvin was able to take his in a concentrated form. I started him off with two acidophilus capsules at every meal for a total of six each day. That was close to a year ago. Irvin gradually reduced the number of capsules as his condition improved. Now he takes them only at the first indication of a canker sore, which he recognizes by a slight tingling at its possible future site. By taking a few capsules at once, Irvin is able to keep the canker sore from developing.

Winifred had been troubled for a great many years with frequent and painful canker sores. She would barely get over one before another one would start. Often she had two or three at a time, and no doctor had ever been able to help her. After a friend suggested that her problem might be caused by a nutritional deficiency, Winifred came to see me.

Analysis of Winifred's dietary intake revealed that she was extremely deficient in the vitamin B complex. She was also lacking in calcium. As soon as I added a high potency B complex, along with some dessicated liver and yeast tablets, and dolomite to her diet, her canker sores got better immediately. They became less frequent, lasted a much shorter time and were not nearly as painful as before. At the end of two months, Winifred no longer had any trouble with them. She still takes her vitamin B complex, dessicated liver, yeast tablets, and dolomite, however, for she has no desire to have her canker sores back again.

Phenomenal benefits for Martha's receding gums surprise dentist

Martha, who is now in her early fifties, had been troubled with a gum ailment since she was a teenager. She had a problem with tartar and plaque accumulation along and under the gum line. This would cause abscesses and pockets where the gums would pull away from her teeth. Martha suffered with bleeding, puffiness, and swelling of the gums. Often her teeth would actually become loose in their sockets.

She went religiously every six months to see her dentist. He would scale and clean her teeth at the gum line and even below to remove the accumulation of tartar and plaque. Several times, minor surgery was necessary to promote healing of the gums.

Last October Martha came to me to see if I could get her through the winter without having a severe cold. She was extremely deficient in vitamin C. I placed her on 4,000 milligrams of vitamin C each day and told her to increase her intake to 500 milligrams every hour at the slightest sign of a cold until the symptoms disappeared. Martha was overjoyed to find that for the first time since she could remember she did not have a bad winter cold. But that was not all: her treatment brought an unexpected fringe benefit.

"My last trip to the dentist was really a surprise to both of us," Martha told me." "He said my gums had become firm and healthy. His instruments would hardly go below the gum line. He thought I must be doing a better job of brushing because my gums looked so much better. I told him I hadn't changed my brushing at all, but I was taking large doses of vitamin C. I also let him know that was the only single change I had made. He just didn't know what to say."

Two other cases show incredible improvement in diseased gum tissue

Dale came to see me about preventing a bad winter cold as so many people do. He was also deficient in vitamin C. I placed him on a supplement of 4,000 milligrams a day. I also told him to take 500 milligrams an hour at the first sign of a cold until all the symptoms disappeared.

Dale had been troubled with bleeding gums since his twenties — a period of more than 30 years. Within two days after starting his vitamin C therapy, his gums stopped bleeding. In one week they healed up completely. He has had no more trouble with them as long as he continues his vitamin C supplementation. He also overcame his major complaint: he has had no more bad winter colds.

Brenda came to me for bleeding gums. Most people who have mouth and gum problems go to their dentist. But Brenda's gums had been bleeding terribly for the past six years. She had already gone to several good dentists, had lots of dental work done, and spent a lot of money. But her gums still bled and gave her trouble.

I knew that Brenda would be deficient in vitamin C, and, of course, she was. I placed her on 5,000 milligrams of vitamin C each day along with some bioflavonoids which are so helpful in strengthening capillary fragility and preventing bleeding.

Within a few days Brenda was able to tell the difference.

She could brush and scrub her teeth vigorously and massage her gums strenuously without getting the slightest tinge of pink on her toothbrush. This was the first time this had happened in more than six years.

Brenda has continued her vitamin C and bioflavonoid supplements faithfully. During the past year her gums have become firm and healthy. She has had no more trouble with them bleeding. Brenda also received a fringe benefit from her treatment: she got through the winter without even a sniffle, much less a cold.

How tooth grinding was stopped in only one night for Judy with unusually quick treatment

One of my patients, Connie, had a five-year-old daughter, Judy, who ground and grated her teeth every night. She had done this for more than a year. Connie had asked her dentist to help Judy, but he knew of nothing that could be done. Connie told me about the problem and I asked her to bring Judy in so I could check her.

Judy was extremely deficient in calcium even though she drank several glasses of milk every day. This is not surprising for many people have trouble in digesting milk and absorbing its calcium into the body. I told Connie to give Judy six dolomite tablets with each meal.

The results were both immediate and absolute. The very first night after Judy took her dolomite tablets, she did not grind or grate her teeth. To experiment, Connie had her skip the dolomite for two days. Judy started right in grinding her teeth again. She takes dolomite every day and has had no recurrence of her problem.

Baby's gas pains completely resolved in less than an hour with outstanding kitchen remedy

One night I got a call from one of my patients, Natalie, about 10:30 p.m. After apologizing for the late call, she told me her ten-month-old daughter, Alexis, had the colic and was not able to sleep. She had been crying and screaming for several hours.

I asked Natalie to have her husband, Bob, come by my house so I could give him a bottle of garlic capsules for her baby. I told her to take three or four of the garlic capsules, slit them open, and spoon the garlic oil into her baby's mouth. If Alexis still had problems, she was to repeat the process half an hour later.

Next day Natalie called me at the office. She said shortly after she gave her daughter the garlic oil, Alexis gave a big burp, smiled, and went straight to sleep. She slept without a sound from midnight until seven o'clock in the morning.

How I solved George's gastritis with an unusual method

George had suffered for a year and a half with gastritis. His abdominal area was sore and tender. He always had indigestion and a severe heartburn after every meal, no matter what he ate. He had gone to four different doctors, including two specialists, but had received no worthwhile results at all. All of them treated George's gastritis with anti-acid preparations which only further reduced the hydrochloric acid content in his stomach. Not one even remotely considered the possibility that George's condition could be caused by a vitamin shortage.

When George came to see me, he had almost had it with doctors, for he'd spent a small fortune on their fees, laboratory tests, and X-rays, all for nothing. I found George to be suffering from a gross vitamin B deficiency. I placed him on a high-potency vitamin B complex (B-100), along with some dessicated liver and yeast tablets. I also asked George to take two garlic capsules with each meal.

In only one week, George's digestion returned to normal. He suffered no more pain, and his gastritis of such long standing had disappeared completely. It has never returned.

How you can get rid of heartburn using this exceptional procedure

The real cause of heartburn is not excess hydrochloric acid in the stomach, as so many people — including a lot of doctors — think, but sugar, and here's why: *sugar is an irritant to the stomach*. It's just that simple. If you could look into your stomach with a gastroscope when you drink a cup of coffee with two teaspoons of sugar in it, you could watch the mucous membrane of your stomach turn fiery red and angry looking as the irritant, sugar, reaches it. Sugar causes an actual burning sensation, not only in the stomach but also in the lower esophagus. That's why you feel as if your heartburn is coming right up in your throat.

So heartburn is caused by sugar, not by excess acid in the stomach. Let me tell you how I discovered that. I used to be overweight and so did a lot of my patients, so I became interested in the problem of obesity. In fact, much of my practice has been directed toward helping fat people reduce. I found that refined white sugar and bleached white flour, as well as the products containing them, are the two main causes of being overweight, although sugar is by far the worse of the two.

At any rate, when I eliminated my refined white sugar intake, I found that my dyspepsia and heartburn disappeared. My fat patients, who also eliminated refined white sugar from their diets, found the same thing to be true. Their stomach problems simply evaporated into thin air. I tell the whole story of this in my book, *Doctor Van Fleet's Amazing New "Non-Glue-Food" Diet.** If you do happen to have a weight problem, then I would heartily recommend that you read it. It has helped untold numbers of fat people to reduce successfully, quickly, effortlessly, and painlessly, for the first time in their lives.

Sugar, and that includes the sugar in doughnuts, sweet rolls, pie, cookies, and cake, as well as soft drinks, irritates the stomach to make it raw and sore. It also decreases the production of hydrochloric acid in the stomach. When hydrochloric acid is decreased, food is not digested properly. It lies in the stomach in an indigestible mass to give you that bloated, full feeling.

What do people do for this? Well, most of them take antiacids which is the worst possible thing they can do, for they now stop the digestive processes completely. The alkaline medication neutralizes what little hydrochloric acid they had working for them and the digestion of protein in their stomachs comes to a complete halt. The acidity in the small intestine is also ad-

---

*James K. Van Fleet, *Doctor Van Fleet's Amazing New "Non-Glue-Food" Diet* (West Nyack, New York, 10994: Parker Publishing Company), 1974.

versely affected, which creates further problems that can even disturb the normal acid-base balance of the blood. Now, constipation is a sure thing since the food cannot be properly digested and assimilated. Of course, the anti-acid does make a person feel better temporarily, and here's why:

Remember that sugar irritates the stomach, making it sore and raw, so now the hydrochloric acid does burn and irritate those raw places. The anti-acid neutralizes the hydrochloric acid that is needed for digestion and makes your stomach feel better temporarily. But the real key to the whole problem is the irritant, sugar.

To increase the production of hydrochloric acid, get rid of your heartburn, and improve your digestion, you need do only three things:

1. Stop eating refined white sugar and all the man-made foods containing it.
2. Take a high potency vitamin B complex like B-50 or B-100 along with some dessicated liver and yeast tablets three times a day. Vitamin B stimulates the production of gastric juices and aids in digestion.
3. Take two or three garlic capsules with each meal.

This simple three-point program works to get rid of dyspepsia and heartburn. Any of my patients with a former digestive disorder can verify this. Let me quote what one of them said to me:

"Doc, for the first time in ten years I don't have to take an anti-acid tablet as soon as I finish eating," Jack says. "I don't get any sign of heartburn or acid stomach any more. Nor do I belch up a lot of gas as I used to. I'm no longer troubled with constipation. Since I stopped eating sugar and started taking vitamin B and garlic, I just haven't had any sign of a pain in the middle."

In case you're wondering, Jack's situation is not unusual at all. It is not the exception to the rule. In fact, it is the rule. It is still amazing to me, even to this day, to see the remarkable recovery people make from their digestive ailments when they follow this simple three-point program. When I hear remarks like "I feel better than I have in five years...I never felt better around my stomach in all my life...my heartburn is completely gone...I haven't had a bellyache in six months," I feel well repaid for my efforts.

How you can miraculously relieve occasional gastric distress

No human body is perfect. There will still be those rare times when your stomach will react even when you're following my three-point program. However, I've found those rare stomach upsets in my patients usually come from a dietary indiscretion — eating something with sugar in it — doughnuts, cookies, a piece of pie, or whatever. Then, too, those holiday dinners on Thanksgiving, Christmas, and other festive occasions like a church supper or a big wedding feast can bring temporary problems to a person.

For those times, I recommend that my patients take papaya tablets. They are available in your health food store and are absolutely superb in settling your upset stomach. I've even been able to eat fiery hot Mexican food, which I love, without any problem as long as I take some papaya tablets along with it.

These tablets are made from the luscious melon-shaped papaya fruit that grows in clusters on short palm trees. It grows only in the tropics where it has been valued as both food and medicine for centuries.

As the fruit ripens, the skin turns from green to an orange yellow. The smooth flesh contains very little fiber and has a characteristic aroma and flavor that is delicately tropical and delicious. The papaya is often called the "medicine tree" because nearly every part of the plant contains some medicinal properties.

Since papaya is so highly perishable and difficult to ship, unless you live in the southern half of Florida or the tropics, chances are you'll have to depend on papaya tablets to solve your occasional gastric upsets. The papaya tablets stimulate your digestive system and get it going again because its enzymes — papain, mylase, and prolase — help digest the proteins and starches you have eaten. Above all, don't resort to those antiacids to take care of an occasional stomach problem. They only upset your system even more. *Papaya and papaya tablets are food* — not drugs like the anti-acids. That's why they can never hurt you.

Sometimes even good natural foods can cause gas when eaten together. For instance, highly acid fruit eaten at the same meal as coarse green vegetables with much fiber and cellulose can cause gassy indigestion. Remember, too, foods like beans, onions, and cabbage can also cause gas on the stomach. But the natural gas of such foods is not the same as the heartburn from sugar. Papaya tablets will work wonders for these temporary problems.

How Frank regained his health after surgery

One of my oldest patients, a 79-year-old man, was unable to hold any solid food on his stomach for months following surgery and a long bout with pneumonia. He had been on a liquid diet and had lost 35 pounds. Frank was thin, weak, worn out, and constantly tired. I had him take small amounts of papaya every hour. Gradually, he gained in strength and was able to eat other foods.

But even after Frank regained his health, he continued to eat papaya. Whenever he ate a high protein food such as meat, fish, or chicken, he would always finish off his meal with papaya. As long as he did this, he had no problem digesting his food. However, if he did not eat papaya at the end of his meal, he always suffered the symptoms that come from incomplete protein digestion.

If you, too, want to keep your digestive system young and functioning properly, then eat papaya or take papaya tablets if you cannot get the fruit itself as we can here in Florida. Papaya may not be the answer to eternal youth that Ponce de Leon was looking for when he discovered Florida, but it could be the next best thing.

How the Case Histories in This Chapter Can Benefit You

Medical textbooks say there is no known cause for canker sores. Theories range from food allergies and deficiencies to environmental factors. Some doctors feel citric acid causes canker sores. Others think they come from a calcium deficiency.

I *do* know that in my practice I have found that a vitamin B complex deficiency, a calcium deficiency, or both, can often be responsible. In many cases, I have been able to clear up canker sores within 48 hours with large doses of the vitamin B complex three to four times daily and from six to eight dolomite tablets — which contains calcium and magnesium — at each meal.

If I cannot find a vitamin B or calcium deficiency, I have the patient take acidophilus capsules or eat some yogurt every day. In stubborn cases, I use all of these — vitamin B to include dessicated liver and yeast tablets, dolomite, yogurt, and acidophilus capsules — to get results. If you have canker sores, this would be your best bet too, since you have no dietary analysis to guide you.

* * *

Vitamin C and the bioflavonoids are not only good for prevention of the common cold, but they are also valuable in the treatment of pyorrhea or pink toothbrush. If you have this problem, or if you have trouble with receding gums, take plenty of vitamin C — 4 or 5,000 milligrams daily — along with the bioflavonoids. A glass of orange juice each day is not enough. You need much more vitamin C than that to keep healthy.

The bioflavonoids can get results in cases of bleeding gums that vitamin C alone cannot do. Their main function is to strengthen capillary fragility and prevent bleeding. They promote healing and benefit the circulatory system.

* * *

Taking calcium in the form of dolomite is the quickest and surest way I know of to stop a person from grinding and grating his or her teeth at night. Even people who drink plenty of milk often are not able to get the amount of calcium they need. Just taking the minimum daily requirement of calcium is no guarantee that it will be absorbed from the digestive tract into the body where it is needed. Calcium is often so poorly utilized by the body that as much as 4 or 5,000 milligrams a day may be needed.

There is no possibility of any danger due to an excess of dolomite, so I always use it as a source of calcium instead of bonemeal. Bonemeal contains phosphorus, and an excess of phosphorus causes the body to lose calcium. Phosphorus is plentifully supplied in a person's regular food, so no supplement of it should ever be necessary.

* * *

Garlic is one of nature's best remedies for gas and indigestion. It cleanses products of putrefaction from the intestinal tract. It also acts as a digestive stimulant. I have found garlic to be highly effective in relieving nausea, vomiting, gas, abdominal distention, and discomfort after meals. It is much better to use than anti-acid preparations to relieve heartburn or indigestion. Here are two good reasons why this is so.

1. *Anti-acids can have a negative effect on human bones, even when taken in small quantities.* Doctor Herta Spencer checked their effect on eleven patients at the Veteran's Administration Hospital at Hines, Illinois, and found that *four popular commercial non-prescription anti-acids caused the loss of calcium from the body.* This could easily lead to osteomalacia, which is a failure of bone to form. The eleven patients had been taking only two tablespoons of the anti-acid preparations three times daily, the recommended dosage on the label.

2. *Anti-acids also slow down and inhibit the digestive process.* They do not help it as garlic does. The stomach contents must be acid before the pyloric valve to the small intestine will open to allow passage of the food from the stomach. If the contents are alkaline or not acid enough, they will remain in the stomach causing further discomfort and delay in the digestive process.

* * *

If you suffer from gastric distress, such as heartburn or indigestion, my three-point program could well give you the relief you're looking for. Let me repeat it here for you.

1. Stop eating refined white sugar and all the man-made foods that contain it.

2. Take a high potency vitamin B complex like B-50 or

B-100 along with some dessicated liver and yeast tablets three times a day.

3. Take two or three garlic capsules with each meal.

And if you really want the best results possible, take four papaya tablets after each meal. You've already seen what papaya did for Frank: it gave him back his good health. It could do the same thing for you.

7

How to Get Rid of Lower Digestive Problems Forever with Strikingly Different and Unique Methods

The three main problems of the lower digestive tract I encounter in my office are constipation, constipation, and constipation. All joking aside, though, constipation is the most prevalent problem of the lower digestive tract people have. Unfortunately, it can lead to a much more serious condition — diverticulitis. Diarrhea is also a common digestive complaint. Other kinds of lower digestive tract ailments I treat in my office are hemorrhoids and colitis. There are still others, but those I have just mentioned are the most common and the ones I will cover in this chapter.

Before I discuss the first case with you, let me give you a few statistics from my own files that will be of interest to you. I have just gone over 50 case histories of lower bowel problems I have treated in my office. All of them had constipation. Improvement was gained in every single case. Before going on my *Three-B Program*, 43 of them strained at the stool all the time. Seven did most of the time. None of them could defecate without difficulty and effort; none of them had a bowel movement every day. Every second or third day, sometimes even longer, was the rule. After going on my *Three-B-Program*, all of them had normal bowel movements each day. Twelve case histories of patients with the opposite complaint — diarrhea — showed their bowel movements were also quickly normalized by essentially the same program.

In short, my Three-B dietary regime helped all my patients who had lower digestive tract problems. It eliminated or relieved 100 percent of their symptoms and in every way normalized their daily bowel activities.

How Betty quickly and easily resolved her digestive problems

Betty came to me to see if I could help her faulty elimination habits. She had an average of only one or two bowel movements a week. Her stools were extremely hard. She had tried every artificial laxative she'd ever heard of or read about. She said none of them had ever given her permanent or lasting relief. Betty also suffered from an extremely bad skin complexion problem.

I found Betty to be extremely deficient in her vitamin B intake. I placed her on my *Three-B Program,* as my patients have come to call it, of the *B* vitamin complex, *Brewer's* yeast — which is also a rich natural source of vitamin B and a bowel stimulant all at the same time — and *unprocessed Bran,* which she was able to get at her local health food store.

Since constipation is also a physical as well as a chemical problem, I asked Betty to avoid the man-made foods that contain so little roughage and residue. I had her replace them with plenty of fresh fruits and vegetables along with stone-ground 100 percent whole wheat bread instead of white bread, natural raw honey instead of refined white sugar, and whole grain cereals that had not been "enriched" or "fortified" with *synthetic* vitamins.

In just two short weeks after she started on her diet, Betty found she was no longer bothered by the constipation that had troubled her for so long. She has not taken a laxative for many months now, nor has she had any recurrence whatever of her former problem. Not only that, her complexion has cleared up completely and her general health has improved so much, she told me the other day she was feeling better than she had in the last 20 years.

"Doc, if I didn't know how old I really was, I'd swear I was back in my twenties," Betty said. "What a wonderful sensation it is to be healthy and regular and feel good again."

Ten years of constipation ended for Sarah with wondrous improvement

Sarah is only 25 years old. She looked to be a good 35 at least, when she came to see me. She had been taking laxatives regularly since she was 15. Sarah had been to doctor after doctor with the same result. They all prescribed some sort of harsh laxative and pushed her out the door with a prescription in her hand. Until she came to see me, Sarah had no idea at all why she was troubled with constipation. Not a single doctor had ever taken the time to tell her, that is, if he even knew.

Before her baby was born, Sarah became very upset and completely disgusted with the way her bowels were acting. She was afraid to give up laxatives for fear they would not function at all. A friend of hers, who'd been troubled with constipation before using my *Three-B-Program,* suggested Sarah come see me as soon as her baby was born.

Sarah was extremely deficient in her vitamin B intake. This, by the way, I have found to be true with every single case of constipation. A vitamin B complex deficiency seems to be the rule in this situation. I placed Sarah on my Three-B Program of vitamin *B* complex, *B*rewer's yeast, and unprocessed *B*ran. I asked her to stop eating all the man-made foods that were causing so much of her problem.

I asked her to replace them with fresh fruits and vegetables, raw if possible, stone-ground 100 percent whole wheat bread instead of white bread, honey in place of refined white sugar for a sweetener, and whole grain cereals from the health food store instead of the boxed cereals she'd been buying in the supermarket. This is a standing operating procedure for all my patients with constipation, to *eat foods that are born — not made* as much as possible.

Sarah made up her mind to go all the way with her new dietary regime. That first night she threw all her old artificial harsh laxatives into the garbage can. She followed my instructions to the letter, and within five days, her bowels were functioning on a normal, regular basis exactly as a healthy person's bowels should function.

As Sarah herself says, "I feel like a brand new person. I used to feel as if I were 65. Now I feel my right age, 25." I can vouch for what she says. Sarah looks her correct age now instead of the way she looked when she first dragged her way into my office.

How you, too, can get rid of constipation using my Three-B Program

I could go on indefinitely with one case history after another about how I've been able to relieve constipation for my patients with the *Three-B Program,* but I think the two examples of Betty and Sarah are enough. Now I want to tell you how you, too, can get rid of your constipation with these unusually easy-to-use methods.

Constipation is caused by two things: one is a lack of chemical stimulus resulting from an insufficient vitamin B intake. The second is a retention of low-residue waste products in the body for too long a time. This is caused primarily by a lack of bulk in the diet. Packaged and processed foods have no bulk and very little residue. Unless the patient has some intestinal anatomical abnormality, I can say without hesitation that a lack of the vitamin B complex and modern, civilized, man-made foods are specifically the exact causes of constipation in every case I have ever handled.

I always have a patient with constipation first of all take the B vitamin complex, brewer's yeast, and two to three tablespoons of *unprocessed* bran each day. The B complex and brewer's yeast, which also contains the B vitamins in their natural state, are important in restoring the strength and tone to the muscles of the digestive tract. Keep in mind that your nerves move the muscles of the bowel, and they will do the job for you only if your vitamin B intake is sufficient. I also ask my patients with constipation to take dessicated liver since it also is a potent natural source of the vitamin B complex.

Unprocessed bran is important to the patient with constipation because it helps absorb moisture and maintain bulk in the digestive system. The retention of moisture is so important, for it keeps the person from suffering unnecessary discomfort from passing dry, hard stools.

Two to three tablespoons of unprocessed bran each day are usually enough. Most of my patients mix the bran with other cereal or use it in hamburger, meat loaf, and so on. All-bran that is available in the supermarket will also provide bulk in your stools, but I by far prefer the unprocessed bran that you can get in the health food store because it has no sugar or other artificial additives in it. Besides, I think it does a better job of furnishing bulk with no possible harshness.

I also ask my patients to avoid the man-made products such as pie, doughnuts, rolls, white bread, and the like. Those that have bleached white flour are the most troublesome since it has no bulk or fiber. They should be replaced by stone-ground 100 percent whole wheat bread and whole grain cereals. Fresh fruit and vegetables — eaten raw if possible — are to be preferred over the canned ones.

To sum it all up, then, you can easily and quickly get over your constipation if you will follow these few simple guidelines:

1. Take a high potency vitamin B complex each day.
2. Take some brewer's yeast each day.
3. Use two or three tablespoons of unprocessed bran every day.
4. Eat fresh fruit and vegetables, raw if possible.
5. Use stone-ground 100 percent whole wheat bread and whole grain cereals.
6. Eat foods that are born, not made.
7. Avoid man-made foods that contain bleached white flour since it has no fiber content at all.

Diarrhea cured with startlingly different procedure

Velma had diarrhea off and on for more years than she cared to remember. Five years before she came to see me, her doctor had put her in the hospital for a gastrointestinal series of barium X-rays. There was no malignancy and he could find nothing to cause her diarrhea, yet she continued to be troubled with it. Her doctor concluded it was nothing more than nerves. She came to see me on the recommendation of a friend, as is so often the case.

I found her to be lacking severely in vitamin B. I placed Velma on my *Three-B program* of vitamin B, brewer's yeast, and unprocessed bran. I also asked her to avoid man-made carbohydrates and processed packaged foods made with refined white sugar and bleached white flour, and to replace them with fresh fruit and vegetables, as well as stone-ground 100 percent whole wheat bread and whole grain cereals.

Velma was a good patient and followed my instructions to the letter. Her recovery was almost instantaneous. Within 48 hours her diarrhea of such long standing ceased completely. She has been following this dietary regime for more than a year now, and her diarrhea has never returned to bother her again.

Sally's ulcerative colitis incredibly healed with natural foods

Sally was 32 years old when she came to see me. She had been troubled with a non-specific ulcerative colitis since she was 15. Her symptoms ranged from bouts of diarrhea with watery mucus and bloody stools to seiges of constipation. She suffered abdominal pain and distention. Even her menstrual periods were upset and disturbed by her colitis. Her treatment had been primarily a bland low-residue diet, mainly of baby foods, mineral oils for her periods of constipation, and a variety of drugs — no less than seven different kinds, Sally said — for her diarrhea.

Sally was deficient in practically every vitamin and mineral, but especially those of the B complex. I placed her on my regular Three-B-Program of vitamin B, brewer's yeast, and unprocessed bran to get her bowel movements back under control. I also had her take a full supplement of all the other vitamins and minerals she was lacking.

Then, very slowly, one food at a time, we gradually got her off her old bland diet onto a more nutritious one. We had to move at an extremely slow pace for fear that too rapid a change would cause her digestive system to react to strange new foods with a seige of diarrhea.

Little by little we made progress. First, white bread was exchanged for stone-ground 100 percent whole wheat bread. Then brown rice took the place of polished white rice. One at a time raw fruits and vegetables replaced the canned baby foods she'd been eating. It took a year to completely switch over from her bland diet to my diet of foods that are born — not made. Today, Sally eats only a bare minimum of man-made packaged or processed foods. She has had no sign of ulcerative colitis since she first started on my dietary program.

Sally's previous doctor had told her that an ulcerative colitis patient's chances of contacting intestinal cancer were about 20 percent higher than those of the average person. He had recommended yearly X-rays to keep close track of the activity and progress of her disease. I urged Sally to do as he asked and to keep going back to him annually for her check-up. She has been back twice now. Her X-rays show that the diseased area is completely healed. There is no ulcer any more and no sign of any abnormal activity. Her doctor has told her that she is completely well.

Diverticulitis gives in to new treatment

Wilson had run the gauntlet of gastro-intestinal specialists before he came to me. He had constant problems with gas, abdominal pain and nausea, as well as an extremely painful rectum. Since he had diarrhea, and because of the painful rectum, his previous doctors had placed him on a low-residue diet. They eliminated raw fruits and vegetables. They did not allow any whole grain bread or whole grain cereals. The result was a diet with stewed meat, soft boiled eggs, dairy products, cooked fruit and soft vegetables, plus refined sweets and starches. But all this only intensified Wilson's problem.

After checking Wilson's dietary intake, I found him to be

extremely deficient in vitamin B. I placed him on my Three-B program of the B vitamin complex, brewer's yeast, and unprocessed bran. I also asked him to avoid the man-made foods containing sugar and starch and to replace them with fresh fruits and vegetables, raw if possible, stone-ground 100 percent whole wheat bread, and whole grain cereals.

Wilson did this. Within a few short weeks all his symptoms of diverticular disease disappeared. I am not saying the intestinal pouches in the colon which were the end result of diverticular disease are gone; that would be impossible. I am saying this diet did eliminate the symptoms that were so distressing to him. Wilson's bowel activity has become normal and he can now live a happy, productive life.

Miscellaneous conditions resolved by this fantastic new diet

Almost any case of lower digestive tract distress can be resolved when the dietary intake is normalized. The natural tendency of the body is to be healthy whenever the proper conditions exist. The lower digestive tract is certainly no exception. Let me cover with you now just briefly two other cases. These two cases were placed on the highly efficient *Three-B-Program* along with the natural foods I recommend for my patients. However, in each one, some additional treatment was necessary as you'll see.

Rectal itching eliminated for Larry

Larry came to me for a constantly itching rectum. He had been bothered with it for as long as he could remember. It was extremely embarrassing to him. When he scratched too hard, it would become sore and on several occasions became infected. He had gone to several doctors for the problem, but the ointments and salves they gave him afforded him only temporary relief.

I placed Larry on my regular *Three-B Program* for intestinal problems, and he responded well. His rectal itching was greatly reduced, but it still bothered him some at the end of the first month of treatment.

At that time, I rechecked Larry's food intake and found he was still taking in far too much sugar in his diet. He had reduced the amount of actual sugar he used as such, but he had failed to take into complete consideration the sugar contained in compound foods. I advised Larry to read the labels on packaged and canned goods more carefully so he could avoid sugar as much as possible. Larry did this, and his rectal itching disappeared completely. He has not been bothered with it now for more than two years.

Hemorrhoids relieved for Kenneth with extraordinary treatment

Kenneth's major complaint when he came to see me was hemorrhoids. They were very painful to him. He had undergone extremely painful surgery twice for them, and he was carefully trying to avoid situations that would aggravate his condition.

After I took down his past history, it became quite apparent to me that Kenneth's hemorrhoids were the result of chronic constipation. He was also deficient in the vitamin B complex so I started him out very slowly and carefully on the *Three-B Program.*

At the end of 30 days, Kenneth's constipation had improved tremendously and he felt much better in general, but his hemorrhoids still hurt and bothered him. I rechecked his food intake and found a gross vitamin C deficiency. Careful questioning of Kenneth revealed that some of the information he gave me the first time was inaccurate.

Based upon the second dietary analysis, I added 3,000 milligrams of vitamin C daily along with some bioflavonoids to Kenneth's diet. This time the pains from his hemorrhoids diminished and became almost negligible. An examination of them 30 days later showed that they were much smaller and not as congested as before.

Although I doubt if his hemorrhoids will ever disappear altogether — after all, there is the scar tissue of two operations to contend with — Kenneth is no longer suffering with them. Not only that, now that his constipation is cleared up, there will be no more hard and compact bowel movements to injure them as before.

Benefits You Can Gain from
the Case Histories in This Chapter

No less an authority than Doctor Lawrence E. Lamb, M.D., heart specialist, and syndicated columnist and lecturer, blames bleached white flour for constipation and many of our digestive problems of modern civilization.

Addressing a Retired Officers' Association convention, Dr. Lamb in effect said this: "Cancer of the colon, which is now a quite common problem in our modern civilization, was unknown over 200 years ago in our society. Today, the highest incidence rate in the world is in New England.

"Why is this? Because we have stopped eating fiber. Our civilized foods have no roughage in them. Instead, we have nice white flour without any fibers in it. African people, in contrast, because their diet contains a large amount of indigestible roughage and fiber, actually don't have the problems we have. An adequate intake of bulk in the diet, which would be a return to the kind of life our forefathers led, would solve our digestive problems. Cereal and other fibers will absorb moisture, maintain bulk in the digestive system, and prevent these problems."*

Why does a low-residue diet of man-made foods produce constipation? Why is a large amount of bulk, roughage, and indigestible fiber needed to prevent constipation? Here's why: waste matter is normally moved along the intestines by waves of muscular contraction. When the bowels are relatively full of waste matter, the muscles surrounding the membrane lining of the intestines need to contract only slightly to move it along. But when waste matter is scanty and compacted, as it is in those eating a highly refined diet of man-made foods, the muscles

---

*The Retired Officer Magazine, 1625 Eye St., N.W. Washington, D.C. 20006, February, 1975.

have to contract with much greater force to create the pressure needed to keep things moving.

It is somewhat like squeezing a tube of toothpaste. When the tube is full or nearly full, only a slight pressure is needed to expel the toothpaste. But when the tube is nearly empty, you have to squeeze and squeeze harder and harder to get the contents out. That's exactly what you do when you strain at the stool. You squeeze harder and harder to get the waste material out.

Occasionally it is difficult for some of my patients to get their bowels back to a normal evacuation cycle rapidly enough to suit them. In those cases, I recommend they add two table-spoons of flaxseed daily to their whole grain cereals for additional bulk.

Above all, do not use mineral oils for a laxative. They rob your body of the fat soluble vitamins A, D, E, and K. Mineral oils also carry calcium and phosphorus out of your digestive tract. However, if you follow the seven guidelines I gave you on page 105, you will never need to use mineral oil. Constipation will become a thing of the past for you.

* * *

Diarrhea as well as constipation responds to my *Three-B-Program*. At first it is hard for people to understand how two completely opposite conditions could respond to the same treatment. Here's why: in cases of constipation, the bran, whole wheat bread, whole grain cereals, fruit and vegetable cellulose and fibers add to the digestive waste, retain moisture, and help to move the waste matter along. In cases of diarrhea, these same food substances absorb water and mucus, thus preventing a runny and watery bowel movement.

* * *

Most doctors treat ulcerative colitis with bland, low-residue diets. Only a few here and there insist on giving their patients natural foods for their conditions. Some enlightened authorities now feel that man-made carbohydrates contribute to ulcerative colitis. Several think the taking of laxatives is often responsible for its beginning. If you do have the problem of ulcerative colitis, study Sally's case carefully. Don't hurry.

Do as she did, changing one food at a time, until little by little, you will have changed your dietary regime to one that has plenty of vitamin B, brewer's yeast, unprocessed bran, and natural foods. Take your time. Easy does it, and success will be yours.

* * *

Diverticulitis is another "civilized" disease. Dr. Neil S. Painter, Senior Surgeon at the Manor House Hospital in London, England, says that diverticular disease is most prevalent in communities where people eat a so-called *civilized* diet that contains primarily products made with refined white sugar and bleached white flour. Such a diet lacks natural roughage and fiber.

Doctor Dennis P. Burkitt, member of the Medical Research Council in London, England, reports that many diseases common in and typical of Western civilization have been shown to be related to the amount of time required for the passage of the intestinal contents through the alimentary canal, as well as the bulk and consistency of the stools.

Studying the dietary habits of African natives convinced Dr. Burkitt that their food, which was heavy with fiber and roughage, kept them from getting cancer of the colon. The doctor also noted that cancer of the colon has become common in Western nations since the introduction of bleached white flour.

Doctor Burkitt says that refined white flour is also largely responsible for such common "civilized" illnesses as heart attacks, appendicitis, diverticular disease of the colon, gall bladder ailments, varicose veins, blood clots in the veins, gastrointestinal hernia, hemorrhoids, and obesity.

He also points out that these diseases are very rare; in fact, they are virtually unknown, in rural Africa where refined white flour is not used. I myself haven't used white flour or white sugar for many years now. I'm sure you can see why.

Actually, diverticulitis is the end result of chronic constipation which comes from those man-made foods made with white flour that lacks raw fiber and roughage. It comes from years of straining at the stool in a constant effort to evacuate the bowels. All this straining causes the muscular walls of the colon to become weakened and separated. The mucous membrane that makes up the inner wall of the intestine forms small pouches that push out here and there as a result of the intracolonic pressure. Eventually definite pockets form that are in a true sense small intestinal hernias.

Diverticulitis may begin slowly with vague digestive symptoms and variable bowel movements. However, as the condition progresses and becomes more chronic, constipation will become the most prominent and striking symptom. It can often be interrupted with attacks of diarrhea as the body tries to cleanse itself of the accumulated toxins and poisons.

In addition, the patient will usually complain of gas on the stomach and bowel, a feeling of distention throughout the abdominal area, nausea, heartburn, and a sore and tender rectum. The person will often say he is unable to completely empty the rectum during a bowel movement. He always feels as if he has more waste to get rid of. If a patient tells me this and has hemorrhoids as well, I am certain he has diverticulitis since these two symptoms indicate a constant straining at the stools.

To prevent yourself from getting diverticulitis or to keep it from getting worse if you already have it, follow the seven guidelines I've listed on page 105 for you. In addition to those, never, and I repeat, *never* strain at the stool. If your stools are so hard and compact they will not move without straining your bowels, then insert a glycerin suppository to soften the fecal mass, but do not strain to get rid of the waste.

8

How to Alleviate
the Aches and Pains of
Arthritis and Rheumatism
Naturally with Incredible Success

Back in Chapter 2 I gave you several examples to show you how cherries could be used to bring relief to sore and aching knees, rheumatism, stiffness in the fingers, arthritis in the arm and shoulder, and gout.

However, cherries are not the only food that can be used to get rid of the aches and pains of arthritis and rheumatism successfully. It is important to remember that no two human bodies are exactly alike in the way they react to treatment. Some respond to one kind of therapy; others are helped by an entirely different kind of treatment.

Over the years, I have found that not only cherries can be of assistance in treating arthritis and rheumatism, but also that many other natural foods can be helpful as well. I will discuss those in this chapter. Before doing so, however, I want to say that no matter what treatment is covered here, you can always supplement it by eating cherries, too. It's for sure they can't hurt you.

How the arthritis in Katherine's knees
was wonderfully healed

When Katherine came to my office, her knees were so stiff and sore that it was extremely difficult for her to get in and out of a car. She even had trouble getting up and down from a chair. She was a meticulous housekeeper who felt her kitchen floor was not thoroughly clean unless she scrubbed it on her hands and knees. This caused her a great deal of pain.

Katherine's previous doctor had diagnosed her condition as arthritis. He had recommended bed rest, a heating pad, and plenty of aspirin to kill the pain. He offered no other treatment. Katherine was completely dissatisfied with this, for she'd been doing those things on her own even before she went to see the doctor. So she came to me.

I found Katherine deficient in pantothenic acid — one of the vitamins of the B complex — and vitamins A, C, and D, as well as calcium. I placed her on a high-potency vitamin B complex, B-50, along with 300 milligrams of pantothenic acid each day. You see, when I detect a deficiency of one of the individual vitamins of the B group, I always give the patient the complete B complex along with that individual B vitamin to insure a balanced intake of vitamin B for the body.

I also gave Katherine 25,000 units of vitamin A, 5,000 milligrams of C, 1,000 units of D, and 2,000 milligrams of calcium in the form of dolomite each day. I asked her to avoid as much as possible the processed and packaged foods that are so high in man-made carbohydrates — refined white sugar and bleached white flour. She replaced them with the natural foods that are born — not made.

Katherine improved remarkably in the first 30 days on her new dietary regime. She has been under my care for more than a year now on a monthly check-up basis and has had no more trouble. She doesn't take aspirin any more at all; her heating pad has long since been stored away in her closet.

Katherine also tells me she has no pain at all in her knees when she scrubs her kitchen floor, although she still gets down on all four's to do it. I don't like her to do that, and I've tried to get her to stop, but this is one bad habit she refuses to break.

How Bill found complete freedom from his troublesome shoulder bursitis

Bill is a telephone lineman who spends 85 percent of his time outside in all kinds of weather. He came to me for bursitis in both shoulders. They were so stiff and sore that he could not raise his arms above his head without tremendous pain; yet, this was the position he found himself in almost all day long.

When Bill came to see me, he was taking a dozen aspirin a day just to keep going. But the aspirin was causing some undesirable side effects, for he'd developed a bad skin rash. He'd also been suffering from a great deal of indigestion with some gastric bleeding.

Bill's dietary intake was terribly deficient in both vitamin C and vitamin P (the bioflavonoids). I placed him on a daily supplement of 6,000 milligrams of vitamin C along with 600 milligrams of the bioflavonoids divided into four equal amounts.

In only 24 hours Bill could tell the difference. The pain and swelling already had begun to subside. In four days, his bursitis was almost gone. At the end of two weeks Bill's shoulders had lost the last vestige of their stiffness. He had complete freedom of movement. He no longer suffered any pain when he raised his arms above his shoulders to work. He still had some tenderness in the muscle tissues around the joints that could be elicited by pressure and palpation, but even this disappeared at the end of 30 days.

Arthritis in hands of secretary-typist relieved in only four months

The young lady who sat across the desk from me was only in her early twenties, but she was no longer able to make a living at her occupation as a secretary-typist because of the agonizing pain in her hands. The joints of her fingers were swollen and stiff with rheumatoid arthritis.

Her previous doctor had given her no hope of recovering from her ailment. He told her she could take aspirin for the pain, and possibly some cortisone shots might help. Maybe even some kind of operation in the future, he said; but for now, he offered her no real hope of any kind of relief.

So Lucy came to see me, not knowing what else to do and hoping I might be able to help her. In a sense, she really had no place left to go or no one else to turn to. Her condition was getting worse, not better. She could no longer earn a living, and no other doctor offered her the slightest hope or recovery.

Lucy was deficient in vitamin A, C, and D, as well as pantothenic acid of the B complex, along with calcium, as so many arthritic patients are. I placed her on a daily supplementation of 30,000 units of vitamin A, 6,000 milligrams of vitamin C, 1,000 units of D, 300 milligrams of pantothenic acid along with a high potency B complex, and 2,000 milligrams of calcium obtained from dolomite.

I also asked Lucy to avoid the man-made processed and packaged foods that contain refined white sugar and bleached white flour, and to replace them with plenty of fresh fruits and vegetables, eaten raw if possible. I also urged her to get enough protein in her diet by eating plenty of dairy products, poultry, fish and meat as well as nuts, whole grain cereals, and stone-ground 100 percent whole wheat bread.

Within two months after Lucy started her treatment, the swelling in her hands had gone down. By the end of the fourth month, there was no visible trace left of her arthritis. She was back on her job full time again. As far as I'm concerned, arthritis is not an incurable disease as so many doctors think, for Lucy's case is only one of many similar cases I've taken care of.

Rheumatism in writer's wrist miraculously cured by pyridoxine

One of my patients is a non-fiction writer of articles for magazines. Max had sprained his right wrist several times. He then developed a chronic rheumatism in his right hand and wrist which was so severe that he was unable to work at his regular profession as a writer without suffering extreme pain. Max does all the first drafts of his manuscripts long hand, and he had reached the point where he could not even hold a pencil in his hand for more than a few minutes at a time.

His regular family doctor gave him a prescription for the pain, but it upset Max's stomach so much that he had to stop taking it. After a second medication did the same, he gave up on drugs. But he still had his sore hand and wrist. A friend suggested calling me, so he did.

I found Max deficient in the usual vitamins and minerals all arthritis patients seem to lack — A, C, D, and calcium.

Besides these, he was not getting enough pyridoxine — one of the B vitamins — in his diet. I also confirmed the pyridoxine deficiency by the QEW Test (Quick Early Warning Test). This showed me this vitamin was one of the major causes of Max's problems.

I placed Max on my usual supplements for arthritis, in his case, 30,000 units of vitamin A, 2,000 milligrams of C, 1,000 units of D, and 2,000 milligrams of calcium in the form of dolomite. Then, specifically to combat the pyridoxine deficiency, I gave him 800 milligrams of B-6 along with a high-potency vitamin B complex.

Max's trouble diminished in just a few days. In only three weeks it disappeared completely. The pyridoxine by itself would no doubt have cleared up Max's hand and wrist eventually, but the other vitamins and calcium, which are so important in treating arthritis and rheumatism, helped too, by speeding up the healing process.

I also asked Max to use the arthritis diet which I mentioned in Katherine's and Lucy's cases to prevent any recurrence of his trouble. I will discuss that diet at the end of this chapter. Max has had no further problems with his hand and wrist.

Fabulous results obtained in arthritis of the neck

For several years Harold suffered with arthritis in the hands and fingers. He used aspirin constantly to help combat the pain. Then he developed arthritis in the neck that was extremely painful. He could not turn his head without tremendous discomfort. Aspirin did not help at all. His doctor suggested a neck cast or collar to limit movement and reduce the pain, but Harold refused. Instead, he came to me.

I was surprised at Harold's dietary analysis. He showed no shortage of vitamins A, C, and D, deficiencies that usually show up in cases of arthritis and rheumatism. However, further questioning of Harold revealed he had been taking large amounts of these three vitamins on his own. He did show a severe deficiency in pantothenic acid, and also a gross deficiency of calcium in his dietary intake.

Harold told me he had cut his calcium intake because he thought too much calcium in his diet was contributing to his arthritis, a mistake many people often make. I gave him a daily supplementation of 2,500 milligrams of calcium in the form of dolomite. I also gave him 300 milligrams of pantothenic acid plus a high potency B complex for proper balance and placed him on my standard arthritis diet.

In exactly two weeks after starting his new dietary regime along with his dolomite, pantothenic acid, and B complex, Harold was able to turn his head without any discomfort in his neck. Shortly after that, to his great joy, the pain disappeared from his hands and fingers and the swelling began to subside. That has been more than six months ago. Harold's symptoms have not returned. His aspirin and other pain killers have all been thrown in the trash can.

Elderly patient survives severe fall without broken bones

One of my patients, Molly, is 82 years old and entirely dependent upon social security and a tiny private pension. She feels she cannot afford all the vitamins I recommend for my arthritis patients, but I do insist that she continue to take dolomite.

The reason for this is that osteomalacia and osteoporosis are among the most common bone ailments found in people in their later years. These are disorders in which there is a gross calcium deficiency in the bones, causing them to become weakened and break easily. Dolomite will help to keep this from happening.

For instance, Molly has had several bad falls in the past several years, but amazingly, she has suffered no broken bones as so often happens with elderly people when they have an accident.

The most recent fall Molly took was quite severe. It could have easily broken the bones of a much younger and healthier person. Molly got up to go to the bathroom during the night, tripped over a small stool, and fell down a flight of stairs from the second to the first floor.

She was quite badly bruised in the hips, back, and shoulders. However, there were no broken bones to be seen anywhere in her X-rays. I feel absolutely certain that if Molly had not been getting plenty of calcium in the form of dolomite, she would have ended up in the hospital with a bad fracture.

Arthritis in knees shows immediate and marked improvement

Several years ago Gene began having trouble with pain and stiffness in both knees. He went to his family doctor who told him he had arthritis. The doctor suggested wearing elastic bandages on his knees, but Gene says these did no good at all. Of course, aspirin was prescribed which did give him some temporary relief from the pain.

As time went on, the pain became more and more severe and Gene could no longer sleep at night even with the aid of aspirin and sleeping pills. Walking became extremely difficult for him, even with a cane. His doctor said he might have to resort to a walker. Going up and down stairs became almost impossible for Gene. He was able to climb stairs only by putting one foot on a step and then pulling his other foot up to that step. Going down was the same slow, laborious process.

Gene was at wit's end about what to do when he heard of my success with arthritis and rheumatism. A friend of his who was under my care had a bony spur on his wrist that was gradually disappearing with treatment. One day he showed it to Gene who remembered how big it used to be. Gene was astounded to see a hard calcium growth dissolving away, so he called me immediately for an appointment.

Gene's dietary analysis revealed the typical deficiencies of an arthritis patient: vitamins A, C, D, pantothenic acid of the B complex, and calcium. I placed Gene on my special arthritis diet, added these supplements, and to his great surprise and amazement, the pain in his knees vanished in only ten days. The stiffness took longer to leave, about three months. But in the end Gene was walking normally again just as if he'd never had arthritis.

How Harriet's backache was resolved by exceptional treatment without painful surgery

Harriet came to my office almost in tears. She had suffered severe back pains for some time and her doctor referred her to an orthopedic surgeon. He told her she needed a back operation because several vertebrae were so badly deteriorated they would have to be fused together.

Harriet dreaded not only the painful surgery, but also the thought of a permanently stiff back to contend with. She was an extremely athletic woman who loved tennis, golf, and bowling. She couldn't think of giving them all up as her doctor had warned she might have to do after the operation.

I X-rayed Harriet's spine in the affected area to determine the exact extent of damage for myself. Three vertebrae had become slightly wedge-shaped and there was damage to the cartilage or the intervertebral discs between them. However, a few months delay in surgery would not be serious. In fact, the orthopedic surgeon had told Harriet to take all the time she wanted to make a decision.

I placed Harriet on my arthritis diet and gave her supplements of A, C, D, the bioflavonoids, pantothenic acid plus the vitamin B complex for balance, and calcium. In addition, I gave her an exercise to use to help stretch the spine. It required the help of her husband.

Harriet was to lace her fingers together behind her head just above her neck. Then Owen was to stand behind her and place his arms under Harriet's upper arms just under the armpits next to her body. Next, Owen was to bring his hands back through those triangles formed on each side of Harriet's body by her arms and place them over Harriet's hands. The final position Owen would assume would be about the same as a wrestler holding a full Nelson on an opponent. Then very slowly Owen was to lift Harriet's body by raising upward with his hands, wrists, and forearms all at the same time.

I told Owen to do this exercise at least four times a day. He was never to jerk, but only to lift Harriet very slowly and gradually until her body was completely off the floor and to hold her there for at least half a minute.

This position allowed Harriet to be suspended in such a way that the entire weight of her body was pulling downward through her spinal column. When done correctly, I told Owen he would hear her vertebrae actually pop as they were pulled apart, with a sound much like the cracking of knuckles.

Within six months Harriet's back pains had completely disappeared. X-rays of her wedged vertebrae showed they were beginning to return to normal. Harriet never returned to the orthopedic surgeon for that back operation.

How the Case Histories in This Chapter Can Benefit You

A deficiency of pantothenic acid, as in Katherine's case, retards the formation of bone while at the same time it induces excessive calcification in the joints. It also calcifies and hardens cartilage. In other words, a shortage of pantothenic acid in the diet lets calcium go from where it's needed in your body to where it's not needed.

New evidence from England definitely ties arthritis to a pantothenic acid deficiency. The English biochemist, Dr. E.C. Barton-Wright, recently said, "I am not claiming I have discovered a permanent cure for arthritis. What I do claim is that we have discovered the cause, the method of control, and the method of prevention."

Although you can get some pantothenic acid from a high-potency vitamin B complex, brewer's yeast, and dessicated liver, it would still be wise to take it as an additional individual supplement to make sure you get enough for therapeutic purposes if you are troubled with arthritis or rheumatism.

I will discuss the other supplements I gave Katherine under the arthritis and rheumatism diet in the last part of this section.

❄ ❄ ❄

One of the most effective treatments I've found for bursitis or rheumatism in the shoulders is vitamin C along with the bioflavonoids. I have also discovered that five to six thousand milligrams of vitamin C daily and at least 600 milligrams of vitamin P or the bioflavonoids at the same time give the best results.

It is always best to divide these amounts into at least three or four equal dosages to be taken at meal times if you use three, or at meal times and bed time if you use four. I personally prefer that a patient take vitamin and mineral supplements four times a day because that keeps the body plentifully supplied throughout an entire 24-hour period.

* * *

Pyridoxine deficiency is one of the most widespread deficiency diseases in the United States. It causes many kinds of muscle and nerve pains and swelling in the joints throughout the body. It is linked to rheumatism and arthritis in some way. Exactly how is not yet completely known or understood.

One of the first signs of a pyridoxine deficiency can be anemia, followed by difficulties with the tendons and ligaments, especially in the hands, along with swelling in the joints there and elsewhere in the body. Women who become depressed while on birth control pills are benefited by taking additional pyridoxine. Also, people who are tense, worried and anxious improve when taking this supplement. Swellings of the hands, feet, around the cheekbones, and other signs of edema indicate a deficiency of pyridoxine.

How to test yourself for pyridoxine deficiency

There is a Quick Early Warning Test (QEW Test) that you can use to test yourself for pyridoxine deficiency just as I used it to double-check the dietary analysis on Max. A Dr. John M. Ellis devised this test. Here's how it works:

Extend your hand with the palm up and the wrist straight. Now bend the first two joints in your fingers until the fingers reach the hand. You do *not* bend the knuckles that are between the back of the hand and the fingers to make a fist. You bend only the first two joints of each finger to touch the hand.

If you cannot bend your finger joints this way, if you cannot reach your hand with them without making a fist, then you no doubt do have a pyridoxine deficiency. If you are a man, you can take from 200 to 600 milligrams daily to correct this. Start with 200 and up the daily intake until your condition begins to improve. Then hold it at that level. If you are a woman, from 300 to 800 milligrams a day would be appropriate. You can find your own level of intake the same way a man does. Don't worry about taking too much. No overdose of pyridoxine is possible. Split your dosages into three or four equal amounts and take them three or four times a day.

* * *

Harold made the mistake so many people make. He thought his arthritis was coming from too much calcium in his diet. So he cut down on his calcium and his arthritis got even worse.

I've had patients come to me with big knotty knuckles and deposits of calcium around the joints — all the deformities of arthritis — who were actually calcium starved because they thought their big sore knuckles and stiff joints were caused by too much calcium in the diet.

Actually, the reverse is true. These calcium deposits are caused by a lack of calcium in the diet along with a disturbance of calcium metabolism. Remember, too, a deficiency of pantothenic acid, not an excess of calcium will cause the excessive calcification of the joints. A shortage of pantothenic acid in the diet lets calcium drift out of the bones where it's needed and go to the joints where it's not needed.

I have never seen a case of arthritis that was caused by getting too much calcium in the diet, and I never will. It is one of the two major minerals (the other one is iron) that almost all Americans are short of. The only major food sources of calcium are milk and milk products because most of the natural calcium in grain products is refined away and lost in the processing. Many of us don't like milk, so the best source of calcium is dolomite. Don't worry about getting too much calcium in food supplements like dolomite. An overdose is impossible.

* * *

If you have a bad back as Harriet had, the exercise I described is one of the best methods I know to correct it and relieve the pain without surgery. It is especially good for relieving the pain that occurs right in the spine between the shoulder blades for so many people. If you have someone around the house who can lift you this way, there is one precaution that should be remembered: have the person lift you with his legs, not with his back. If he is the same height, it is best to have him stand on a stable footstool about six inches in height.

If you are alone, then fix a pipe about one quarter inch in diameter in a doorway or some other convenient place. It should be high enough you cannot reach the floor when you hang from it by your hands. Use a small stool to reach the bar and do your stretching exercises. Do this exercise several times a day, and you will accomplish the same thing as if someone were lifting you, except that it will not exert a pull on the cervical or neck vertebrae. Also, it will take just a little longer to get the desired results.

How you, too, can avoid the aches and pains of arthritis and rheumatism with this marvelous diet

This is the basic diet I use for all my patients who have some kind of arthritis or rheumatism. The actual amounts of vitamins and minerals used vary with each individual and are based on my analysis of the dietary intake.

First of all, I ask the patient to cut out all man-made packaged and processed foods that contain refined white sugar and bleached white flour. There is an overwhelming body of scientific evidence to prove that white sugar and white flour are responsible for many chronic ailments, including arthritis, rheumatism, coronary thrombosis, atherosclerosis, cancer of the colon, gall bladder disease, diverticulitis, hemorrhoids, and obesity. After these foods are eliminated along with saturated fats, I ask the patient to refrain from using tobacco and alcohol and to follow this diet:

1. Fresh fruits and vegetables, eaten raw if possible. Many patients find a blender or a grinder extremely useful.

2. Plenty of protein foods to include milk, cheese, and other dairy products, poultry, meat, and fish. Processed meats containing sodium nitrate and sodium nitrite should be avoided.

3. Whole grain cereals, nuts, stone-ground 100 percent whole wheat bread.

4. Unsaturated cold-pressed fats and oils such as sunflower, safflower, corn, cottonseed, soybean, peanut oil. Usually cold-pressed oils are not sold in supermarkets, but only in health food stores.

5. Following vitamins and minerals on a daily basis:

   a. Vitamin A 25 to 50 thousand units.

   b. High potency vitamin B complex, such as B-50 or B-100, dessicated liver, and yeast tablets three times a day.

   c. Pantothenic acid, a B vitamin, 100 to 300 milligrams.

   d. Pyridoxine, a B vitamin, 200 to 800 milligrams.

   e. Vitamin C, 2,000 to 8,000 milligrams.

   f. Vitamin D, 1,000 units.

   g. Vitamin P (bioflavonoids) 600 milligrams. Used especially for cases of bursitis or rheumatism in the shoulders.

   h. Calcium, 1,000 to 3,000 milligrams from dolomite.

If you take these vitamins and minerals for your rheumatism or arthritis, start with the lower figures and gradually work up to the higher ones or to whatever level of intake you get results. When taking pyridoxine or pantothenic acid, always be sure to take a B complex along with them. Taking one of the B vitamins always increases the body's demand for the entire complex.

It is important in a diet for arthritis to get natural foods as much as possible. This means foods that have not been packaged or processed or changed by cooking, drying, storage, or preservation. Fruits and vegetables should be fresh and ripe, grown by organic methods, free from residues of pesticides and fertilizers, if such are available.

The last thing I ask my patients to do is get off aspirin, pain killing drugs, and all corticosteroid medications as soon as feasible so their bodies will have a better chance to heal themselves naturally without outside interference. These kinds of medications simply delay the healing process.

9

How to Get Rid of Headaches, Insomnia and "Plain Old Nerves" with These New and Remarkable Healing Methods

These three ailments — headaches, insomnia, and "plain old nerves" — drive most doctors up the wall in frustration and despair. Trying to find the cause of a headache as well as the cure for it is an extremely difficult task for the average practitioner. Insomnia presents just as much of a problem. "Plain old nerves" is a label a lot of doctors hang on a patient's nervous complaints when they can find nothing else to blame the person's vague and abstract symptoms on. And whenever a doctor can't find the cause or the cure for a person's problems, he'll say it's imaginary...it's all in the mind...and push the patient out the door with a prescription of some sort so he can get on to the next person who's *really* sick.

But I know from experience that headaches, insomnia, and plain old nerves are conditions that are as real as sin to the patient. For instance, when I was a child, I watched my own mother suffer in misery for years and years with "sick" headaches simply because no doctor could find the cause or the cure for them. Today I know she had severe migraines, and I also know there is relief for such headache victims. They are not hopeless cases.

I am thankful every day I practice that I use the dietary approach to disease to find out what is causing a person's problems. Unless I did, I'm sure I'd be completely in the dark, too. But with dietary analysis, I've learned that almost all cases of headache, insomnia, and plain old nerves are coming from a food deficiency of some sort.

There will be exceptions, of course. The possible problems in one's life — money, marriage, job, and so on — can cause these three conditions to develop, too. But I've also found that a dietary deficiency is even more likely to exist here; for when a person is down in the dumps, has the blues, and is feeling depressed, his appetite is never up to par and he simply doesn't eat the way he should.

How Mary got rid of her hypoglycemic headaches with unusually easy-to-use methods

Mary had been suffering for several years with headaches that occurred nearly every morning an hour or two after she got to work at her job as a receptionist. My examination showed that her sugar consumption was far too high, while at the same time, her protein and calcium intakes were far too low.

Detailed questioning of Mary revealed that on the mornings she went to work, she was grabbing a couple of doughnuts and a cup of coffee with two teaspoons of sugar at *Mister Donut* since she did not take time to cook breakfast at home. Those were the mornings she always had her headaches. But on Saturdays and Sundays when she did not have to hurry to get to work, Mary would have a slow leisurely breakfast of steak, ham, sausage, or bacon and eggs. On these mornings she had no sign of a headache at all.

I pointed out to Mary that her heavy consumption of sugar every morning — two doughnuts and coffee heavily laden with sugar — was causing her blood sugar to act like a yo-yo due to her over-sensitive pancreas. You see, in those two doughnuts she was getting 12 teaspoons of sugar — the average glazed doughnut contains six teaspoons of sugar — plus two more in her coffee for a total of 14 teaspoons of sugar on the way to work each morning. Then as soon as she got settled down at her desk, it was another cup of coffee with two more teaspoons of sugar and a cigarette.

Now when too much sugar comes into the blood stream all

at once, as it did after Mary's doughnuts and coffee each morning an over-sensitive pancreas secretes too much insulin to metabolize that sugar, and then, unfortunately, the blood sugar falls below normal. No wonder Mary was having her miserable nervous morning headaches.

I asked Mary to avoid all the man-made foods containing refined white sugar and to eat a good balanced diet of fresh fruits and vegetables so she could get plenty of energy from natural sugars and starches. I especially asked her to avoid those breakfasts of doughnuts and heavily sugared coffee and to replace them with a high protein breakfast of meat — steak, bacon, ham, sausage — and eggs. Then to make up for her calcium shortage, which was also contributing to her nervous headaches, I asked her to take dolomite every day with each meal and before going to bed.

Mary could hardly believe that such a simple remedy as this could solve her problems and cure her headaches. So she wavered back and forth. She would follow my instructions one day only to violate them the next. But her penalty was always the same: nervous morning headaches.

Finally, she decided to "kick the sugar habit for good," as she put it. When she did, she found she no longer had to put up with those morning headaches for the first time in many years. She was able to rid herself of them permanently. Today, Mary absolutely refuses to touch refined white sugar, or to eat any foods containing man-made carbohydrates. She gets all the natural carbohydrates she needs from fresh fruits, fresh vegetables, and raw honey. These three supply her with all the energy she needs.

Headaches, and a great many other ailments, too, caused by low blood sugar are much more common than most people realize. I will discuss hypoglycemia more fully in Chapter 12 for you.

Incredible new solution for the misery of migraines

Alma had been plagued with migraine headaches for as long as she could remember. They would awaken her at four or five in the morning several times a week. As Alma told me, she had tried every remedy anyone had ever suggested to her — strong coffee, ice packs, hot towels, aspirin, brandy, and so on — but nothing ever seemed to do her much good. A friend told her how I'd been able to help her sinus headaches, so Alma called me.

I found that she was suffering from a severe vitamin B deficiency. I gave her a high potency vitamin B complex (B-50) some brewer's yeast, and dessicated liver tablets. I also gave her 800 milligrams of pyridoxine (vitamin B-6) and 2,000 milligrams of niacin (vitamin B-3) in the form of nicotinic acid for these reasons:

I have found pyridoxine to be extremely valuable in the treatment of headaches, chronic fatigue, tension, stress, and other nervous conditions. I have also found that niacin in the form of nicotinic acid is beneficial in relieving the cranial vascular constriction that so often accompanies migraine headaches. No overdose is possible with any of these vitamins.

I also asked Alma to avoid refined white sugar and the foods containing it, for I have found that most migraine sufferers also have a problem with low blood sugar. Although this condition may not be the total cause of migraine headaches, low blood sugar does seem to be a major contributing factor for it tends to intensify them.

Alma responded wonderfully to her treatment. At the end of only one week she was completely relieved of her headaches. Three months have now gone by and her migraines have never come back. And as long as she continues to take her vitamin B supplements and limits her sugar intake, I do not expect them to return.

Another example of migraine solved by unusual methods

Nora came to me with the same problem: migraine headaches. She had suffered with them for 15 years, ever since she was 14 years old. She averaged three or four of them every month. She had all the major symptoms of severe migraine:

spots floating in front of her eyes, obstructing her vision, flashes of light, nausea and vomiting, followed by severe pounding, usually one-sided, severe headaches. As Nora said, it always felt as if her head was going to split right in two from the pulsation and throbbing of the blood vessels in her brain.

I found Nora to be not only deficient in vitamin B, but also short in vitamin C. She also had a deficiency in both calcium and iron. I gave her a high-potency vitamin B supplement along with some dessicated liver and yeast tablets. I also had her take 3,000 milligrams of vitamin C each day as well as some dolomite and an iron supplement.

Since starting her treatment, Nora has had only two migraines, although both were comparatively minor, she said. They were much less severe than she'd been used to. Both of these happened in a one-week period of time when Nora stopped taking her vitamins just out of curiosity to see if they were really helping her. She has never done this again; she needed no more convincing.

How Noland's headaches were quickly eliminated by unorthodox methods

Noland was troubled with severe, skull-pounding headaches that seemed to come out of nowhere for absolutely no logical reason. Sometimes he would awaken in the morning with one. At other times they would develop during the day or in the evening. We could not tie them down to a dietary indiscretion as in Mary's case. Nor did the kind of day Noland had appear to be influential. As he said, "I've had some of my most miserable headaches on my best days at the office as well as on my worst days."

The analysis of Noland's dietary intake revealed he was suffering from a vitamin E deficiency. Frankly, I could not tie Noland's lack of vitamin E to his headaches, for I'd never seen a case like that before. But no doubt about it, Noland was short in vitamin E, so I asked him to take 1,200 units of vitamin E each day, divided up into four equal amounts, one for each meal and one at bed time.

Within a short time, Noland's headaches disappeared. As long as he continues his vitamin E supplementation, they do not return. For an understanding of the physiology in this case, turn to the last part of the chapter where I discuss it on page 138.

Sinus headaches disappear as if by magic with this unique treatment

Al came to me suffering with severe sinus headaches. These had bothered him for a long time, and each winter they seemed to be getting worse. He had tried every sinus remedy he'd seen advertised on TV, but none of them had done him any good. In fact, several of them definitely made his problem worse, he said. Finally, Al reached the point he could no longer stand his condition the way it was so he came to see me.

I found that Al was deficient in vitamins A, C, and D as well as zinc. I immediately placed him on a daily supplement of 30,000 units of vitamin A, 6,000 milligrams of C, 1,000 units of D, and 30 milligrams of zinc.

Although Al had suffered with his nasal congestion and sinus headaches for many years, his condition improved even more slowly than either of us liked. You see, even though I'm a doctor and I realize how the body needs a reasonable amount of time to heal itself, I'm still human too, and I'm just as anxious as the patient to see his condition improve.

So in Al's case, since his ailment was so deeply entrenched, I reasoned this way. If I could figure out some way to get the vitamins and zinc Al needed directly to the affected tissue, I knew we could clear up his nasal and sinus congestion much more rapidly and get rid of his headaches for him.

For instance, I knew that vitamin E taken orally will speed up the healing of burns. But I also knew that vitamin E applied directly to burned tissues will heal them even faster. All I needed to do was devise some method of getting the vitamins and zinc Al needed up into his sinuses so they would relieve the congestion.

So here's what we did. I had Al get a cool spray humidifier. He filled it with boiled water almost up to the full mark. Next I had him add some liquid vitamins A, C, and D. Then we crushed a couple dozen zinc tablets in the solution.

Al would breathe in this vitamin and zinc water mist through his nose at least every hour for ten minutes or so. Fortunately, his job permitted him to do that during his working hours, too. In just six days, Al's sinus congestion of so many years cleared up. When it did, his sinus headaches disappeared, too.

Al continues to take his vitamin A, C, and D supplements orally along with his zinc, but he also uses his humidifier with the vitamin and zinc water mist several times a day as a preventive measure. He has had no sign of his condition returning, but as he says, he doesn't want it back. Al would rather put up with the slight inconvenience of using a humidifier rather than suffer with sinus headaches again.

How Teresa solved her insomnia overnight without sleeping pills

Teresa was extremely nervous and jumpy and had been taking sleeping pills for quite some time. However, her body had evidently adapted itself to them for they were no longer effective for her. After hearing a TV program criticizing various sleeping pills, cold remedies, and heartburn medicines as being worthless, she decided to take a radically different approach to her problem of insomnia.

My physical examination of Teresa revealed no specific difficulties that could be causing her insomnia. Nor was I able to find any psychological problem in her life that could be a contributing factor. But the dietary analysis was a completely different story. Teresa was deficient in calcium, magnesium, and zinc, all of which are necessary for a calm and properly functioning nervous system.

I placed Teresa on dolomite for her calcium and magnesium deficiency (2,000 milligrams of calcium and 1,000 milligrams of magnesium) and gave her 30 milligrams of zinc all on a daily basis. Zinc is a natural tranquilizer for the nervous system. I also asked her to take six tablets of calcium *lactate* before going to bed along with a glass of warm milk. The calcium in calcium lactate is quickly and easily assimilated by the body and I have found it is the best form of calcium to take for insomnia.

The very first night Teresa slept better than she ever had with sleeping pills. During the following weeks her body completely eliminated the harmful effects of the drugs in her sleeping tablets which helped her natural remedy of calcium, magnesium, and zinc to become even more effective. Teresa no longer has one bit of trouble sleeping. She says she's never slept this well since she was a little girl.

How Dick successfully got rid of insomnia caused by poor circulation

Most cases of insomnia are due to the mineral deficiencies of calcium, magnesium, and zinc as in Teresa's case. However, Dick's insomnia was caused by a completely different set of circumstances so I want to tell you about his case specifically.

About four years ago when he was only 57, Dick came to me because he was unable to get a good night's sleep. His arms and legs constantly became numb and went to sleep on him. They became so painful that they would wake him up several times a night. His doctor at that time blamed Dick's problem on poor circulation — a result of old age, he said. However, he could offer no relief of any sort to Dick.

My examination of Dick showed that his other doctor had been correct in his diagnosis that the cause was poor circulation. But he was wrong on the second part. It was not due to "old age," but due instead to a lack of vitamin E.

Since Dick's blood pressure was normal and he had no history of rheumatic heart disease, I placed him on 1,200 units of vitamin E each day immediately. Had there been a problem of high blood pressure or a history of rheumatic heart disease, I would have begun his vitamin E consumption at a much lower level — probably 100 units a day — and built it up more slowly over a longer period of time.

Dick responded magnificently to the vitamin E therapy. He has never had any more problems with his arms or legs going to sleep on him at night. The vitamin E cleared up his circulatory problem completely. As Dick himself says, "I sleep like a baby, Doc. Don't know what it is to have insomnia any more, thanks to you."

How Arnold made a fantastic recovery from nervous depression

Arnold had been hospitalized for a nervous breakdown before he came to see me. He had fallen into a deep depression, had lost all ambition and interest in life and was extremely nervous, unable to relax or sleep at night. He could not concentrate on his work. At the time Arnold was attending Southwestern Missouri State College in Springfield, Missouri, but he had to withdraw because of his condition.

His doctor told Arnold there was nothing physically wrong with him, that it was all in his head. A few weeks after he left the hospital, Arnold came to my office. I found that he was suffering from a severe B complex deficiency, as well as a shortage of calcium.

I placed Arnold on a high-potency vitamin B complex (B-100) along with dessicated liver and brewer's yeast tablets to correct his vitamin B deficiency. I also gave him dolomite to solve his calcium shortage. I asked him to avoid refined white sugar as much as possible for it is notorious as a cause of nervous problems.

In only one week, Arnold began to improve rapidly. He became calmer and lost his nervousness. He could relax and sleep at night. In less than three months Arnold was a completely changed person. He was planning on going back to college for the next semester.

How Dora magically overcame her extreme nervous tension

When Dora came to see me, she was so nervous that no part of her body was ever completely still or at rest. She was constantly tapping her fingers, biting her nails, scratching her head, or crossing and uncrossing her legs. She said she was extremely impatient with her husband and children and snapped at them for no good reason whatever. She was always restless, easily annoyed, grouchy and irritable without any good reason. The slightest noise was almost unbearable, and she felt as if she were looking at the world through a film or a haze.

"I haven't had a good night's sleep in a year," she said. "I wake up at the slightest noise and then I can't get back to sleep. Don't you dare say there's nothing wrong with me like my last doctor did. I know something's wrong and I want you to find out what it is so you can help me."

I immediately suspected Dora's problem to be a severe calcium deficiency, for one of the first major signs of a calcium shortage is extreme nervousness. Without calcium, the nerves cannot send messages properly. Muscles become tense and cannot relax. In children, this nervousness from a calcium shortage will show up in unpleasant dispositions, temper tantrums over nothing, and constant whimpering or crying spells.

Dietary analysis not only confirmed my suspicions of a calcium shortage, but it also revealed that Dora needed more vitamin B and D. Of course, I should have suspected that, too, for both the B complex — especially B-1 — and vitamin D are necessary for proper calcium absorption and assimilation.

I placed Dora on dolomite each day to correct her calcium deficiency. I also asked her to take five calcium lactate tablets with a glass of warm milk before going to bed to help her insomnia. I gave her a high potency vitamin B complex (B-100) with dessicated liver and yeast tablets along with 1,000 units of vitamin D each day to correct her vitamin deficiencies.

In only a few short days Dora became calm and serene. She was like a new woman. Her problems caused by a vitamin and mineral shortage disappeared completely. Today she feels fit and full of vigorous health and vitality.

How You Can Benefit from the
Case Histories in This Chapter

If you get a headache, just before meals, when a meal is overdue, or within an hour or so after eating a heavy sugary meal just as Mary did, chances are your problem is of hypoglycemic origin. No doubt your pancreas is oversensitive and releases too much insulin into the blood stream at the slightest hint of excess sugar in it. When that happens, your blood sugar then falls far too low and you get a hypoglycemic headache.

The cure for this is not more sugar in the diet, as so many

people think. In fact, heavy consumption of refined white sugar in coffee, candy, sweet rolls, doughnuts, pie, cake, ice cream, and so on at this time will only make the condition worse. You'll get a temporary relief, perhaps, but the heavy and sudden onslaught of man-made carbohydrates into your blood stream starts the vicious cycle all over again.

You can stabilize your blood sugar at the proper level only when you eat natural carbohydrates and proteins and avoid the man-made foods that are the trouble-makers. Proteins and natural carbohydrates digest more slowly and the natural sugars from their digestion move into your blood stream at a much slower pace than refined white sugar. The movement of these natural sugars is slow enough to keep from triggering your pancreas in the release of too much insulin under normal circumstances. However, when you are already troubled with hypoglycemia, it will take time for your oversensitive pancreas to adjust to your new diet of foods that are born — not made, so give it a fair chance to work for you.

* * *

Low blood sugar and a vitamin B complex deficiency both seem to contribute to migraine headaches. Niacin, one of the B vitamins, especially seems to be a vital factor. I tell all my patients who are being treated for migraine to take 50 milligrams of niacin in the form of nicotinic acid *immediately* if they feel even the slightest hint of a migraine coming on. You see, migraine headaches always seem to be associated with a constriction of the blood vessels in the brain. Niacin helps dilate those constricted blood vessels. If 50 milligrams of nicotinic acid do not create a flush, then I tell them to take another dose of 50 which should be enough.

Don't be frightened by the intense flushing action. Your face may turn beet red, burn, prickle, and itch for a short while, not more than 15 minutes on the average. This is not dangerous. It is only an indication that your circulation has been stirred up. One function of the vitamin B complex is to help your body metabolize or burn up the sugars and starches in your body for energy purposes. A deficiency of this vitamin upsets your sugar metabolism and contributes to the low blood sugar so often found in migraines.

Although Noland's headaches were not truly migraine, they were still vascular in nature. Here's what I mean by that. Whenever there is insufficient oxygen in the blood stream and in the tissues, they will suffer. Waste products are not removed properly. Energy cannot be supplied to the tissues.

For example, if you were to place a tourniquet on your arm, you would cut down or eliminate completely the flow of blood with its oxygen to your forearm and hand. Now if you were to clench and unclench your fist rapidly, it would be only a short time before you would be screaming in agony because the waste products are not being removed and new energy or food supply to the muscles has been cut off.

This was what was happening to Noland. Because he lacked vitamin E, his tissues, especially his brain, were not receiving the proper blood supply. The oxygen to his brain was reduced, and, therefore, severe headaches would develop. Had his job been muscular rather than mental, then his problem could have shown up in his muscles.

You see, vitamin E increases the supply of oxygen to all the tissues. Not only that, it helps them use oxygen more efficiently. In Noland's case, the vitamin E supplement he took increased the oxygenation of his brain tissues and relieved his headaches.

Noland also received a major fringe benefit from his vitamin E supplementation. He tells me he is much quicker, sharper and more alert than ever before. He doesn't tire as fast mentally. He also has noticed that he can make decisions much faster now and without undue hesitation. All this from vitamin E and an increased blood supply to the brain where it was so vitally needed.

* * *

Using a cool spray humidifier to inhale a water mist containing liquid vitamins A, C, and D along with zinc is better than all the sinus medicines you've seen advertised on TV put together. Vitamin A is essential for the health of your mucous membranes. So is vitamin D. The two of them together are required to keep the mucous linings of your nasal, bronchial, and lung cavities moist so they can function properly. Vitamin

C is needed to heal infections while zinc has been found to speed up the healing process.

I've also found this vitamin and zinc spray to be of great assistance in clearing up the nasal congestion of colds, allergies, hay fever, and the like. It's also helpful in cases of bronchitis and asthma. Just don't expect it to perform an overnight miracle for you although occasionally that will happen. Give it a few days to work and you'll be more than pleased with the results you get.

* * *

I did not cover any specific cases of tension headaches for you, but I would like to give you a few procedures you can use to get rid of them. Tension headaches are caused by muscular strain or some nervous situation which causes you to hold yourself tight and tense over a period of time. For instance, suppose you were driving home on a dangerous, icy highway in bumper-to-bumper traffic during the five o'clock rush hour. By the time you got home safely, your neck would feel as if it had been in a vise and your arms would be ready to fall off. The same thing happens when you're in a dentist's chair. Innumerable situations can cause the nervous headache that comes from muscular stress, strain and tension.

The solution? Massage is excellent therapy. Buy a good vibrator, the kind that fits on the back of your hand. Have your husband or wife massage your neck and shoulders for five minutes or so. You'll forget you ever had a headache.

Another good method to use is neck traction. The lifting exercise — not the bar exercise — I gave you back in Chapter 8 on page 121 is good to relieve the headaches of muscle tension. Or while you're lying on the bed getting your neck massaged, have your partner use this simple neck exercise to help your headache.

Have him cup one hand under your chin and the other hand behind the base of your skull. Then have him pull slowly and smoothly as far as it will go. Keep your neck muscles completely relaxed while he's doing this. Don't worry about injury. It won't happen as long as he doesn't jerk your head. All he has to do is make the movement smooth and slow. Easy does it.

If you have insomnia, your best bet is to do as Teresa did. Take dolomite to be sure you get enough calcium and magnesium for your nervous system to function normally. Also take 30 milligrams of zinc daily for zinc is nature's own tranquilizer. Then at bed time, take half a dozen calcium *lactate* tablets along with a glass of warm milk. Milk also contains calcium. This procedure is much safer and more effective than the bromides used in sleeping pills. Some of my patients add a teaspoon of raw honey to their milk, which is good since honey is itself a natural sedative.

If milk is not for you, take your calcium lactate tablets and drink a cup of chamomile tea. This is an herbal tea that will calm the nerves, relax the body, and sooth the stomach. You can find it in any good health food store. Some of my patients who do not like milk tell me the chamomile tea works wonderfully for them.

A warm bath, a good massage, a walk before bedtime — all these will leave you relaxed and they will help, too. However, I do know when you're upset emotionally or when you have pressing problems on your mind, I don't care how healthy your body is, you won't be able to go to sleep immediately.

I don't intend to make this a book on psychology or psychiatry, but I can say this much about emotional problems that can be helpful to you: forget about yesterday and tomorrow. Let those two days take care of themselves. You can't do anything about either one of them. *Live only in the ever-present now,* and a lot of the problems that are keeping you awake will disappear immediately.

* * *

I have found calcium to be outstanding in its ability to relieve nervous symptoms more quickly than perhaps anything else. For example, if a person's muscles become unexpectedly and suddenly weak and shaky...if his hands tremble when he's exerting himself...if he feels weak and trembly in the legs...usually all he needs is more calcium. A great many times a patient's irregular pulse and palpitations of the heart can be restored to normal in a matter of hours with calcium.

Or take a woman for instance. Sometimes she will break down and cry for no apparent reason at all that a man can see. And she won't be able to give a good reason why either except that her nerves are jagged and on edge. A lot of doctors will say that she's neurotic, that there's nothing wrong with her, that it's all in her head, but I know that 99 times out of 100, she's not neurotic at all. She's short of calcium, and that's what her body is crying for.

* * *

So if your problem is "plain old nerves" and your doctor insists you're not really sick, do this: take some calcium in the form of dolomite every day. Add 30 milligrams of zinc on a daily basis. For vitamins, take at least a high potency B complex like B-50 or B-100 along with some dessicated liver and brewer's yeast as well as 1,000 units of vitamin D. And it wouldn't hurt to take some extra A, C, and E either. Cut down your refined white sugar and bleached white flour consumption. Increase your consumption of foods that are born — not made. So help me, if you don't feel better and get rid of your plain old nerves, well, I'll throw in the towel, but then, I know that you will feel better.

10

How to Have a Glowing, Youthful and Radiant Complexion with These Unusually Easy-to-Use Methods

The average general practitioner is as hard pressed to find the cause and cure of skin conditions as he is with headaches, insomnia, and plain old nerves. He does not like to take care of skin problems at all unless he is a specialist in that field.

But I never feel that way. I really enjoy seeing a patient with a skin ailment come into my office, for I know I can help that person. I know I can make him well. There is no doubt or any question whatever about that in my mind, and here's why...

Skin problems reflect a vital food deficiency of some sort

I don't have to play guessing games to find out what's causing my patient's skin condition. I don't have to try one salve or ointment after another only to be disappointed and frustrated in the end. All I need to do is determine the dietary deficiency the patient has, be it an essential vitamin, mineral, or a combination of these. Once I know the cause of my patient's condition from my dietary analysis of his food intake, then I know what to do to cure it.

For instance, I have had cases of acne and eczema that were completely healed with vitamin A after other doctors have called the conditions hopeless. Other patients have needed the vitamin B complex, while still others were deficient in vitamin E. Then there have been those cases deficient in all three of these essential vitamins. Some have required additional zinc to relieve their conditions; and acidophilus capsules have sometimes been the answer, as you've seen in earlier chapters.

All my patients with skin conditions have been the tough cases other doctors have given up on. I cannot recall a single person with acne, eczema, psoriasis, shingles, or what have you, who had not gone to at least one and usually two or three other doctors before he or she came to see me. As I said in the beginning, most patients with chronic ailments come to a chiropractor only as a last resort. And that is especially true of persons with skin problems.

How Paula's severe acne and deep facial scars were healed with spectacular results

I have achieved some absolutely spectacular results in my practice curing so-called hopeless skin eruptions and infections with vitamin A. Let me tell you about one of those cases now.

When Paula was only 13, her face became severely infected with acne. Her mother was extremely worried about the effect on Paula's physical health, as well as the possible traumatic psychological changes to her developing teenage personality.

They went to several skin specialists who tried everything they could think of to use as a remedy, but nothing ever helped Paula's mother even asked their family doctor to examine Paula for a possible vitamin or mineral deficiency since she felt that might be the cause of her daughter's troubles. However, their doctor assured them that vitamins had nothing at all to do with Paula's skin problems.

It was several years later while Paula was attending Southwest Missouri State College in Springfield, Missouri, that her roommate told her how she too had been troubled with severe acne back in high school before she came to see me. As she told Paula, I had cleared up her acne completely and her face had become quite normal again without leaving any scars.

Encouraged by this, Paula and her mother came to my office. Her physical examination and my dietary analysis of her food intake revealed a gross vitamin A deficiency. I immediately placed her on 30,000 units of vitamin A each day and gave her some vitamin A oil to apply directly to the lesions. I also asked Paula to avoid refined white sugar and bleached white flour as well as any of the man-made foods containing them.

In only three weeks Paula had no more *new* eruptions on her face for the first time since she'd been 13 years old six years ago. She was extremely elated and optimistic about this development. Her face was quite badly pitted and scarred, so much so that it was not until the third month of treatment we realized the pitted places were gradually filling in and the scars were slowly disappearing. Today, all those pits and scars are gone and Paula has a normal, healthy-looking complexion.

How Charlie received astounding relief from skin infection in only three short days

When Charlie came to me, he had an extremely bad infection on his face and neck. He told me no drug or medication had been able to give him any relief. During the past year he'd been to six different doctors for a total of more than 30 visits, but none of them had helped him at all. In fact, Charlie said most of the salves and ointments they'd used had only made his condition worse.

My dietary analysis of Charlie's food intake showed he was suffering from a severe shortage of vitamin A. I immediately placed him on a daily dosage of 35,000 units. I also gave him vitamin A oil to apply directly to the affected areas. In only three days the infection that had troubled Charlie for more than a year was beginning to clear up. At the end of one week it was gone altogether and his face looks perfectly clear and healthy again.

University professor of chemistry gets phenomenal improvement in severe skin condition

Elbert had a bad skin rash on both sides of his nose. He went to a skin specialist who gave him a prescription for an ointment similar to one given to people who have poison oak. It worked quite well for him, but after several months of continued use it became apparent to Elbert that whenever he stopped using the ointment, the rash would reappear. He finally realized he was treating the symptoms rather than getting to the cause of his problem, so he stopped using the ointment and came to my office.

I found that Elbert was severely lacking in vitamin A. I gave him a daily dosage of 50,000 units along with some vitamin A oil to use locally, and his rash disappeared in less than a week. He has not had any more trouble with it at all. We since have lowered his intake to 25,000 units a day. Elbert does not mind taking vitamin A continually. He does not classify it as a drug or a chemical, but simply as a food that he needs every day.

"Chemicals are for the chemist, not for the human body," Elbert says. And he ought to know what he's talking about. After all, he's a university professor and an expert in the field of chemistry.

"Emotional" skin problem remarkably cured by vitamin A

Gail had been troubled by a skin eruption that occurred on the inside of both arms around the elbow joints. She went to a dermatologist who told her it was probably due to some deep-seated nervous problem or emotional disturbance, no doubt brought on by strain, tension, worry or overwork. In spite of this diagnosis, he still recommended an antibiotic ointment for her to use.

However, Gail felt if her condition was emotional or nervous in nature, she would have the rash on other parts of her body too. The ointment her skin specialist prescribed did little to help her, so Gail finally came to see me, although with some misgiving. You see, she was a registered nurse, and all her medical background and training had led her to distrust doctors of chiropractic and to view them with suspicion.

In spite of this, Gail was an excellent patient. When I discovered that her condition was due to a vitamin A deficiency, she accepted my diagnosis and followed my directions without argument or question. I placed her on 35,000 units of vitamin A each day along with some vitamin A oil to put on the irritated areas.

Gail got rid of her "emotional" skin condition in less than a month when her dietary deficiency was corrected. Her skin eruption has not returned, and it won't just so long as she continues to take her vitamin supplement to prevent any further shortage.

After two years, Mildred finally gains relief from "incurable" skin condition

A little over two years ago, Mildred developed an itching skin rash under one of her rings. She took the ring off, assuming that this would make the itching stop and cure the rash. Unfortunately, this did not happen.

A year later, the itching was much worse and the skin rash had spread. The rash, diagnosed as eczema by several prominent and well-known dermatologists in a large midwestern city, now covered her entire hand. It could not be stopped in spite of all the expensive ointments and salves her skin specialists prescribed for her.

"Not only did the intense itching keep me awake at nights, but I was also extremely embarrassed by the way my hand looked," Mildred said. "I no longer could go out in public without wearing gloves no matter how hot the weather was. I was almost on the verge of a nervous breakdown for fear the rash might go up my arm and perhaps onto my body. I was afraid to touch myself anywhere with that hand. I had no idea where or when, if ever, it was going to stop, and neither did any of those high-priced skin specialists."

Mildred heard of me from a friend of hers whom I'd helped with a skin problem. She finally gave up on the dermatologists and traveled over 200 miles to see me. I quickly diagnosed her problem to be a vitamin B complex deficiency. I immediately placed her on a high potency B complex (B-100) along with some dessicated liver and yeast tablets, all to be taken four times a day.

In less than a month the itching stopped completely and the rash started to regress. In a little over two months, it disappeared altogether. Mildred was overjoyed. She looked at the results as a miracle, but as I told her, it wasn't a miracle at all. It was just nature at work. All we had to do was supply her body with the proper nutrition. When we did that, nature took care of the rest.

After 20 years of suffering, seborrheic dermatitis yields to unprecedented treatment

Ella was 42 years old when she came to my office the first time. She had suffered with seborrheic dermatitis since she'd been 21, a period of more than 20 years. The dermatitis was primarily along her facial hairline, but it also extended down to her eyebrows and along both sides of her nose. She wore her hair in bangs all the time to try and cover her forehead as much as possible. The condition was greatly embarrassing to her.

During those 20 years of suffering, Ella had consulted 12 dermatologists. Some of them told her she had a glandular condition while others said it was her nerves. They did agree on one point, however: they all said it was incurable and that she would just have to live with her problem.

Ella told me there wasn't anything on the market that she hadn't tried: shampoos of all kinds, creams, salves, ointments, lotions, rinses, hot olive oil, and so on. Nothing ever helped. The closest she ever came to any success whatever was a prescription with sulphur in it. This did remove the dry scales of her dermatitis, but it left her skin with red blotches on it for several days afterward.

I found Ella to be extremely deficient not only in the entire vitamin B complex but especially so in one of its components, PABA, or para-aminobenzoic acid. I placed her on a high potency B complex (B-100) and asked her to take three tablets a day, one with each meal. I also had her take an additional supplement of 100 milligram PABA tablets, also one with each meal for a total of three a day. I should mention here that there are no precautions to be observed with PABA. Since it is a vitamin it is a food, not a drug, and is therefore harmless at all levels of intake. It causes no bad side effects.

After 20 years of suffering, Ella could hardly believe the results herself. She was delighted, for in only three weeks her dermatitis vanished. It disappeared completely and has never returned. That has been more than five years ago now. During the past five years, Ella has enjoyed a clear and healthy complexion without the slightest sign of her former seborrheic dermatitis. Of course, she still takes her vitamin B complex and PABA supplements, but at a reduced level.

Patient receives marked benefits from unusual treatment of eczema

Sandra had put up with eczema on her hands for more than five years before she came to see me. Although she was only 27 years old, her hands were like those of an old woman who'd done laundry by hand all her life. They were swollen, fiery red and cracked everywhere. They hurt and itched all the time.

She too had been to several skin specialists, but to no avail. Every one of them had used salves and ointments that did nothing to help her. Not a single one of them had ever considered the possibility that Sandra's eczema could have a nutritional basis.

I examined Sandra and found that she was badly lacking in her intake of the vitamin B complex. I put her on a high potency supplement of vitamin B (B-100) along with some dessicated liver and yeast tablets. She took these supplements three times a day. In only five short days her eczema was gone.

Sandra could hardly believe it. Her hands were clean and clear. They were no longer cracked, red, and swollen. The itching had stopped completely and the pain was gone. Her hands were small and beautiful again for the first time in more than five years.

Sandra continues to take her vitamin supplements without question, for she realizes that vitamin B is a food, not a medicine. Once in a while, if she forgets to take her vitamins, her hands will swell up and break out again; but as soon as she gets back on her supplements, her eczema will disappear, usually by the next day.

"Sandpaper" complexion responds beautifully to unique methods

Lois came to me for a very peculiar skin problem: she had a skin rash that left her face very rough. It actually felt just like sandpaper to the touch. She had tried everything on it, but nothing she used would make it go away.

My dietary diagnosis revealed that Lois had a vitamin E deficiency. I placed her on 1,200 units of vitamin E each day and gave her some vitamin E oil to use on her face several times a day. Within only three days her skin began to feel smooth again. At the end of one week it was perfectly clear and as soft as a baby's.

Psoriasis is not an incurable disease after all

Dan had been cursed with psoriasis for the past eight years. If you have ever had psoriasis, you know it is one of the most annoying and unsightly skin conditions you can be troubled with. You also know that it is considered to be incurable by almost all doctors.

Half a dozen leading dermatologists had told Dan it was hereditary or caused by nerves and that there was no known permanent cure. After all kinds of salves, ointments, baths, lights, and lots of money down the drain, Dan resigned himself to his condition. He figured no one could help him.

Then luckily he heard of me through a friend. I found that Dan had a severe vitamin E deficiency. I placed him on 1,500 units each day and gave him some vitamin E oil to use on the affected areas.

In three weeks, Dan noticed that his psoriasis was disappearing. It had vanished completely from his left leg and his hands were almost clear. At the end of six weeks, there was no sign left of his condition.

Itching scalp marvelously healed after patient gives up all hope

Roy had been bothered for some time with an itching scalp. As a result of much scratching, it had become infected and he had several large scabs and open sores when he came to my office.

My dietary analysis revealed that Roy had a vitamin E deficiency. I placed him on 1,200 units each day. In addition, I gave him some vitamin E oil to use on his scalp. I told him to use it like a hair tonic and to apply it liberally each night before going to bed.

The first night Roy used the vitamin E oil the itching stopped within an hour. In ten days all the sores had healed, the scabs were gone, and the itching had not returned. Roy still takes his vitamin E capsules each day. He also massages the vitamin E oil into his scalp twice a week to prevent the condition from coming back.

Six-year skin rash
amazingly disappears at last

Willis had been bothered with a red, itching skin rash like measles on his chest for six years. As is true with almost all my skin patients, he had gone to several skin specialists and had taken many remedies without receiving anything more than just temporary relief.

Willis also had a vitamin E deficiency. I gave him vitamin E oil to use externally on the affected area and 800 units to be taken orally each day. This cleared up his problem in less than a month. The lesions disappeared completely and the itching is gone, too.

Vitamin E oil works wonders in topical skin use

Let me just briefly tell you about some of the results I've gained from the use of vitamin E oil externally in several cases:

1. Carla had been troubled with an unsightly skin ailment on both arms that numerous doctors had diagnosed as a kind of psoriasis. She had tried every kind of possible treatment her doctors suggested, but nothing ever helped.

I had her use vitamin E oil on the affected areas. With just two applications the itching stopped in only one day. She continued using it twice daily for one month and her condition was gone completely. She can now wear short-sleeved dresses and blouses without worry or embarrassment about her arms.

2. Kelly had a sore on his leg about the size of a quarter that would not heal. Every time it was bumped or scraped it would bleed. After four months of this Kelly came to see me. I had him use vitamin E oil on it. The sore began to heal immediately and was gone at the end of two weeks.

3. A neighbor of mine, Imogene, upset a boiling pan of water on her hand. When I saw her two days later, it was badly blistered, painful and fiery red. She was deeply worried about permanent disfiguration of her hand and rightly so. I gave her some vitamin E oil to use on her hand. Within a week it had healed completely without leaving a single trace of a scar.

4. My wife's hairdresser, Florence, is allergic to permanent wave solution. Her hands were constantly broken out with a painful rash. I gave her a bottle of vitamin E oil to use on them. Within a week her hands had cleared up beautifully. She now uses it all the time as a hand lotion to prevent the condition from developing again.

5. I have used vitamin E successfully in case after case to rid patients of painful and troublesome warts. A good way to apply it to the wart is to soak a band-aid with the oil and place it over the wart. The wart will not go away overnight. I have had cases where three to four months have gone by before they finally disappeared. Patience and time are required.

Three case histories show how little-known mineral solves skin problems safely and quickly

Let me quickly tell you how zinc can often work wonders for troublesome skin conditions.

1. For more than three years Vivian suffered with acne. I found her to be deficient in zinc. Now after only one month of taking 30 milligrams of zinc each day her face is beautifully clear, and her friends are astonished by the results.

2. Victor had been troubled with acne since he was 14 years old. It got worse for him over the years despite a variety

of treatments he tried. He was 23 when he came to see me. I put him on 30 milligrams of zinc each day. His face cleared up completely in only three short weeks.

3. Riva was always bothered with a dandruff problem. Her scalp would begin to itch and flake about three days after washing her hair. After I placed her on 30 milligrams of zinc each day, this problem stopped. She is no longer bothered by dandruff or an itching scalp even if she goes a week or more without shampooing her hair.

Horrible eczema of hands yields to unconventional treatment

I want to give you one example to show you how a patient required vitamins A, E, the B complex, and zinc to clear up a skin condition. This will help you to better understand why the *shotgun method* of treatment I recommend for you later on is feasible and sensible.

About three years ago, I saw one of the severest skin problems I've ever seen in my office. When Nina came to me, her hands were dark red in color and had a rash from the tips of her fingers clear up to her wrists. Her hands were so dry that the slightest pressure would cause the skin to crack open and bleed.

Nina told me the condition had started a year before she came to my office. At first the condition had been limited to her palms. She went to a dermatologist, and his diagnosis was a form of eczema. She was given a prescription for a cortisone ointment to be used every night. The doctor told her to wear white cotton gloves while she slept. At the end of four months with this treatment, the condition had spread from her palms down to the ends of her fingers and up to her wrists.

I found Nina to be deficient in vitamins A, B, and E, as well as in the mineral, zinc. I placed her on 50,000 units of A, a high potency B complex (B-100) to be taken four times a day along with some dessicated liver and yeast tablets, 1,200 units of vitamin E, and 30 milligrams of zinc. I also gave Nina some vitamin E oil to use on her hands.

At the end of two months, Nina's hands were completely

healed. Needless to say, she is continuing to take her vitamin and mineral supplements without question.

How You Can Have a Glowing, Youthful and Radiant Complexion with These Easy-To-Use Methods

In this chapter, I've given you just a few of the many cases of skin problems I've solved in my practice. If I were to cover all of them, I could more than fill this entire book. So I've tried to be selective to show you how skin conditions can be caused by a shortage of vitamins A, B, E, the mineral, zinc, or a combination of all of these. Vitamin E can also be used externally on the affected areas in either a cream or an oil, as well as taken orally.

I would like to stress that almost every skin ailment I've ever seen (except for the fungus of athlete's foot) has been due to a dietary deficiency of some sort. If a bacterial infection is present, it is always secondary. It will disappear when the affected area is supplied with the proper vitamins and minerals missing from your diet.

Why do dermatologists and skin specialists use the chemical method to try and cure skin conditions rather than the dietary approach? Because that is the orthodox way; that is the way they have been trained. But all that a chemical salve or ointment can do is contain or control (more or less) the secondary bacterial invasion. A salve or ointment can never correct the dietary deficiency, and that's what must be done if the condition is ever to be cured.

❊ ❊ ❊

Now since I cannot make a dietary diagnosis of your food intake for you, how can you benefit from this chapter? You can use the *shotgun method* to get results. By this I mean that you can take all the vitamins and minerals I've discussed here to cure your skin condition or to improve your complexion if you have no specific problem to correct.

For instance, if I were you, I would take the following vitamins and minerals for my skin on a *daily* basis.

1. Vitamin A, 30,000 to 50,000 units. Oil from vitamin A capsules can also be applied directly to the affected areas.
2. A high potency vitamin B complex such as B-100 (three to four tablets each day) along with dessicated liver and yeast tablets.
3. Vitamin E, 800 to 1,200 units. Vitamin E oil can also be used locally on the skin.
4. Zinc, 10 milligrams three times a day for a total of 30 milligrams.
5. Acidophilus capsules, two with each meal.

The *shotgun method* is not a waste of money. Those vitamins and minerals that might not be specifically needed to cure your particular skin condition could easily prevent some other chronic diseased condition from developing.

You'd also be wise to observe the following guidelines I've touched on in previous chapters for other reasons:

1. Stop eating refined white sugar, bleached white flour, and all the man-made foods containing them. Avoid all processed and packaged foods as much as possible.

2. Eat foods that are born — not made, especially fresh fruit and fresh vegetables, for your sources of natural carbohydrate. You do not need refined white sugar for energy. Natural carbohydrates, including raw honey for sweetening, furnish all the energy you need.

3. Eat your fruits and vegetables raw whenever possible. Never cook them unless it is absolutely necessary to do so. Raw fruits and vegetables are much more nutritious for you than those that are cooked.

4. Use unsaturated cold-pressed vegetable oils and fats instead of the saturated animal ones. *These are also needed for a clear skin and healthy hair.*

5. Eat stone-ground 100 percent whole wheat bread, whole grain cereals, and two or three tablespoons of *unprocessed* bran each day.

6. Get plenty of protein in your diet each day: lean meat,

fish, poultry, cheese, eggs and milk. Avoid processed meats that contain sodium nitrate and sodium nitrite.

If you do happen to have seborrheic dermatitis, you should most definitely avoid refined white sugar. It has been found both clinically and in the research laboratory that sugar is involved in producing this disease. And once seborrheic dermatitis has a foothold, sugar consumption prolongs it and prevents healing.

* * *

You can purchase natural cosmetics by mail order or at most health food stores, such as a vitamin A gel, a vitamin E skin cream, or vitamin E oil to help your complexion. A vitamin E soap that also contains vitamins A and D is useful too. These items are perfectly all right to use. In fact, I heartily recommend them. They will not create a rash as many medicinal salves and ointments so often do.

I always keep a bottle of vitamin E oil handy in our house to use in case of minor burns, cuts or scratches. It helps the skin heal rapidly and prevents redness and scarring.

11

How to Keep
Your Heart and Circulation
Remarkably Young and Vital

Do you have high blood pressure? Are you troubled with varicose veins, phlebitis, Buerger's disease, thrombosis, skin ulcers on your ankles or lower legs? Do you suffer from cramps in your legs after walking only a short distance? Are you excessively short of breath after mild exercise? Do you have too rapid a pulse rate even when you're resting? Do your legs ache, pain and cramp at night? If you have any of these problems, then this chapter will be beneficial to you. If you've been fortunate enough to escape these ailments so far, this chapter will still help you, for you'll learn what you can do to prevent these conditions from happening to you.

I want to show you how you can correct the damage already done or how to keep any further problems from developing. I want to let you know how to strengthen your heart and blood vessels, even if you've never had any cardiovascular problems before. With the correct food supplements and the proper care, you can keep your heart and circulation remarkably young and vital indefinitely. The person does not live whose circulatory system cannot be helped in some way by the proper vitamins, mineral and food supplements.

How your cardiovascular system works

Your heart weighs about 12 ounces, is reddish-brown in color, and is shaped more like a pear than a heart. Although the heart has four chambers, it is actually two pumps. One pump moves blood to the lungs where carbon dioxide and other waste substances are exchanged for fresh oxygen. The other pump, the other side of your heart, moves the blood throughout the body to supply all your tissues with oxygen.

Although it seems as if your heart never rests, actually it does. It takes less than half a second for the left side of the heart to contract and push blood out into the body. Then it rests for half a second before the next muscular contraction. When you are asleep, your heart rests even longer between contractions, for your pulse rate slows down by 15 to 20 beats per minute.

The average person's body has between 60 and 70,000 *miles* of blood vessels. Each pound of excess fat adds about 200 more *miles* of tiny blood vessels — the capillaries. If you are only 20 pounds overweight, you have added 4,000 miles of blood vessels to your cardiovascular system. This increases the work the heart must do.

The arteries carry the blood to all parts of your body. They help the heart move the blood along. They expand each time the heart pumps and contract each time it rests between beats. This lets the blood move in a steady, even flow to your body's extremities.

Once in the farthest parts of the body away from your heart, the fingers and toes, the blood must return through the veins. It follows the course of least resistance on its way back to the heart by moving from the smaller blood vessels to the larger ones. Valves in the larger veins keep the blood from going back toward the fingers and toes again. The veins are also helped in this task by the muscles in your arms and legs, for muscular activity aids in moving the blood back to the heart.

How I lowered Joe's blood pressure with this unusually easy-to-use method

Joe came to me suffering with constant headaches, ringing in the ears and dizziness. He had a sensation of a distinct pounding and throbbing in his head every time his heart beat My physical exam revealed Joe had a blood pressure of 195 over

100. He was also 50 pounds overweight. I advised him to lose weight first of all since every pound of extra fat raises the blood pressure, often by a full point or more. I also asked Joe to take three garlic capsules with each meal.

Three months later I checked Joe again. Unfortunately, he had not lost a single pound, but his blood pressure had dropped to 130 over 80, a very normal figure. All his troublesome symptoms of headache, ringing in the ears, and dizziness had also disappeared. I double-checked with Joe to see if he had made any other changes in his diet or his lifestyle. He had not, but he had taken the garlic every day without fail, just as I had asked him to do.

This was the first case in which I recommended garlic capsules for high blood pressure. I was extremely gratified at the results and have used garlic in many cases since then with extremely favorable results.

Orville's blood pressure improved with this extraordinary method, too

Orville also came to me for high blood pressure. His systolic reading was 180, his diastolic 95. His readings were not as high as Joe's, but he was not as old as Joe, nor was he overweight either. Orville complained of constant headaches and excessive fatigue.

I placed Orville on garlic therapy, three capsules with each meal for a total of nine each day. I asked him to check back with me in a month. At that time, I found his blood pressure was down to 160 over 85. At the end of the second month, the systolic had dropped to 145; the diastolic was still 85. On Orville's third check-up, three months after he'd started his garlic treatment, his blood pressure had gone down to 125 over 80. It has remained there ever since. He no longer suffers with headaches or fatigue — these symptoms are gone completely.

No other food supplement, vitamin, or mineral was used in Orville's case. No other change was made in his diet. Garlic was the only "medicine" he took. Orville also gained a fringe benefit from the garlic: he had suffered with chronic diarrhea for several years that he did not tell me about initially. About ten days after he started using garlic, it disappeared and has never come back.

How Joyce got rid of her high blood pressure and regained her health

When Joyce first came to see me, her blood pressure was 230 over 120 and she was 60 pounds overweight. She was troubled with constant headaches, dizziness, ringing in the ears and excessive fatigue. She could not do her routine household chores without wearing out completely.

Joyce had been taking tranquilizers for nearly three months to quiet her nerves without any relief whatsoever. She was also terribly constipated, so much so that she had a bowel movement only once or twice a week, and then only with the aid of a harsh laxative.

I could find no vertebral misalignment severe enough to cause Joyce's troubles, so I turned my attention to her dietary habits. I found she was lacking in calcium and vitamin B. I placed Joyce on dolomite to get rid of her calcium shortage and a high potency B complex along with some dessicated liver and brewer's yeast to take care of her vitamin B deficiency. Vitamin B is also important in getting rid of the symptoms of excessive fatigue. It acts as a pick-up to restore a person's pep and energy. To help her get rid of her constipation, I also had her take several tablespoons of *unprocessed* bran each day.

To get Joyce's weight down to normal and help reduce her high blood pressure all at the same time, I asked her to stop her consumption of fat-causing "glue foods," the man-made packaged and processed foods containing bleached white flour and refined white sugar. I recommended that she use my "non-glue-food" diet to regain her health. I discuss this marvelously safe and sane weight-reducing diet in my book, *Doctor Van Fleet's Amazing New "Non-Glue-Food" Diet.** If you have a

---

*James K. Van Fleet, *Doctor Van Fleet's Amazing New "Non-Glue-Food" Diet.* (West Nyack, New York, Parker Publishing Company, Inc), 1974 .

weight problem, please read it. It will show you how to lose all your excess fat quickly, easily and permanently, no matter how much you weigh now. I also had Joyce take three garlic capsules with each meal for a total of nine each day to help in lowering her blood pressure.

At the end of eight months, Joyce was like a new woman. She had made almost a complete recovery. Her blood pressure had dropped to 125 over 85, a quite acceptable figure. Joyce was no longer troubled with any of the symptoms of hypertension with which she had previously suffered: headache, dizziness, and ringing in the ears.

Her constipation had completely disappeared and she was having normal bowel movements every day. She got rid of 54 of her 60 pounds of excess weight and was now able to do all her housework without any physical discomfort or undue fatigue. She also had stopped taking tranquilizers at the end of the first month under my care.

Joyce obtained all these excellent results by taking the proper vitamins and minerals and by following my non-glue-food diet to get rid of her excess weight. Would you look at this as an amazing recovery? Joyce certainly did, but to tell you the truth I really expected it, for I've seen it happen so many times before when a deathly sick and discouraged person comes to me for help.

How I was able to help Lloyd's heart trouble with natural means

Lloyd was 52 years old when I first saw him in my office. He had angina and severe shortness of breath. He was completely discouraged with his health. In fact, he told me he had no more desire to go on unless I could help him live a normal life again. Lloyd could not walk even two blocks without constantly stopping to rest because of the pain in his chest. He had already suffered several coronary attacks; he was using nitroglycerin as medication.

I immediately suspected Lloyd was deficient in vitamin E. My analysis of his diet confirmed my suspicions. Since Lloyd's blood pressure and pulse rate were normal and he had no past history of a rheumatic heart ailment, I placed him on 1,200 units of vitamin E a day, 400 units with each meal. I also asked him to avoid white sugar and white flour as much as possible since both of these are known to be at least partially responsible for heart disease.

All this took place more than 15 years ago. Today, Lloyd is 67. He has not suffered an attack of angina since he first came to see me. He retired two years ago but until then, he put in a full work schedule at his office five days a week. He still walks at least two miles each day. Since he retired, Lloyd goes hunting and fishing a lot. He plays 18 holes of golf once or twice a week. He is physically very active and lives a completely full, healthy and happy life.

How a cardiac invalid was cured by exceptional measures

Five years ago when Brad came to me, he was in such poor health he had very little hope of living much longer. He had already suffered seven heart attacks. Four of them had hospitalized him for several weeks at a time. One attack had resulted in an obstruction of one of the branches of the coronary artery, a true coronary thrombosis. Brad could not do any physical work at all. After a couple of minutes of exertion of any sort he would have to stop and rest. He could not walk a block without pain in the chest and gasping for breath.

My analysis of Brad's food intake showed a marked vitamin E deficiency, which I already suspected. Almost every single case of cardiovascular disease I've seen has been deficient in vitamin E. A few will require other treatment; I'll tell you about a couple of them in a minute. I placed Brad on 400 units of vitamin E three times a day for a total of 1,200 units.

Vitamin E often works so miraculously that it is hard to believe the superb results it obtains. Within only three months, Brad had forgotten he ever had a cardiac attack or that he'd been troubled with heart disease. He now mows his lawn, a job that takes nearly three hours since it's a big lawn. He walks a mile each day, sleeps well at night, and has no sign of pain in his chest or shortness of breath any more. Vitamin E turned him from a cardiac invalid into a normal, healthy person.

Mike's heart responds magnificently to different treatment

Mike suffered from a rapid pulse and occasional palpitations of the heart. He had a pulse rate of 94 instead of the normal 72 beats per minute, so his heart was not able to relax and rest enough between beats.

My analysis of Mike's diet showed him to be very deficient in his intake of calcium, magnesium and potassium. I corrected this by giving him dolomite and potassium tablets every day. When I added these minerals to his diet, Mike's pulse rate slowed down to normal in only three days. His heart irregularities also ceased. Mike has had no further problems of any sort with his heart or his pulse rate.

Rose gets spectacular results with her heart ailment

Rose had been troubled with attacks of what is called "auricular fibrillation" for years. Her pulse would become completely irregular with a beat as high as 150 to 160 per minute. She had been to many doctors over the years, but none of them had ever been able to help her. Most of them told her it was just "plain old nerves." They usually gave her sedatives which did nothing at all to help. As Rose told me, "They just dulled my mind and made me feel stupid."

When Rose came to my office, she was 59 years old. She had given up the idea of ever getting any relief. She actually came to me only as a last resort, not really expecting any results, but hoping I might somehow be able to help her. I examined Rose and found her to be suffering from a severe vitamin B complex deficiency.

I placed her on a high potency B complex (B-100) to be taken three times a day along with dessicated liver and brewer's yeast tablets. I asked Rose to cut down her intake of refined white sugar. White sugar steals the body's vitamin B reserves. It draws them away from areas where they are vitally needed, in Rose's case, the heart.

Rose has been under my care for six months now and has had no further attacks of auricular fibrillation. Her pulse rate has become strong and steady. It is a regular and normal 72 beats per minute. All signs of her previous problem have completely vanished.

How I quickly cured Caroline's aching legs

Caroline suffered a great deal with constantly aching legs. She worked on a factory production line and was on her feet eight hours a day. By the end of the working day, her ankles would be swollen from congested blood. The calves of her legs ached horribly. They were so sore and tender she could hardly bear to touch them. Many times she could barely make it to her car, for her legs would cramp so badly she couldn't walk. She could relieve the cramps only by vigorously massaging the calves of her legs, which caused her intense pain.

When I examined Caroline, I found her to be extremely deficient in vitamin E, as I knew she would be. Since she had no previous rheumatic heart problems and her blood pressure was normal, I placed her on 1,600 units of vitamin E daily to be taken in four equal amounts of 400 units each time. This was a slightly higher dosage than I normally use on a patient in the beginning, but since Caroline was unable to do a different job at the factory and her work kept her from sitting down, I knew it was necessary.

I was not at all optimistic about her case in view of her working conditions. However, I was wrong. Caroline responded marvelously. In only one month, the vitamin E improved her circulation so much that her legs stopped bothering her altogether. Her ankles no longer swelled, nor did the calves of her legs become painful, even after working all day long. Caroline told me she was now able to do her housework at home and take care of her two sons, ages ten and twelve, without any trouble as well as hold down her full-time job.

How Arline got rid of her leg cramps
with this safe, easy method

Arline had trouble with leg cramps for more than six years. Several previous doctors had diagnosed her condition to be intermittent claudication. This is a spasm of the arteries causing muscular cramping in the legs with severe pain and limping. It is brought about by a decreased blood supply to the legs. Her former doctors' diagnoses were correct; however, their treatments were not. Various medications, drugs and pills had been prescribed and used with no relief at all.

My dietary diagnosis showed that Arline needed more vitamin E. I put her on 1,200 units of vitamin E each day. Within only one month, she received so much relief she told me it was almost like a miracle. For the first time in more than six years, Arline can walk long distances with no pain whatever. She has not had a single sign of a cramp or any pain in her leg since starting her vitamin E supplementation.

Paul's phlebitis responds superbly
in only one short week

Paul called me first from his home. He said he was sure he had a large blood clot in one of the big veins in his left leg. He was afraid to call a medical doctor since he felt sure the doctor would want to operate, and he didn't want that if he could avoid it. However, he was afraid of the clot moving, reaching his heart, and causing a coronary occlusion. I told Paul to stay in bed and not even get up to go to the bathroom until I could examine him.

My physical examination of Paul revealed that a huge blood clot had formed in the femoral vein in his left thigh. The flesh around the clot was red, hot, inflamed and sore. The vein itself stood out under the skin like a rope. It, too, was extremely tender to the touch.

I asked Paul to remain in bed and gave him 2,400 units of vitamin E at once. I told him to continue taking vitamin E, 2,400 units daily, for a week before we made any other decision about what to do. We had not long to wait. At the end of only

24 hours, the clot had begun to disappear. The vein in the thigh softened and lost its rope-like quality. The area around the vein improved too, and was no longer hot and inflamed. At the end of one week, the clot and inflammation were completely gone. Paul was back on his feet without having to resort to surgery, thanks to vitamin E.

Bedfast patient recovers in short order with vitamin E

Shortly after Paul's experience, I had a call from Scott, who'd been bedfast for three months with a severe case of phlebitis. Paul had told him of my success in his own case, so Scott wanted to see me.

Because of the length of time Scott had already had phlebitis, I was not absolutely certain of a full recovery. As with Paul, I used 2,400 units of vitamin E a day. I was deeply gratified when Scott recovered too: in less than two weeks, he was up and on his feet, walking around the house. At the end of only one month of treatment, he had recovered completely.

Scott is now very active again, in fact, more so than before he had phlebitis. He still takes vitamin E, 1,200 units a day. He is 73 years old, walks for an hour every morning, and helps at the Senior Citizens Club in the afternoon three days a week. His leg has never bothered him again. Scott tells me he's more energetic and feels better at 73 than his own children, who are in their forties.

Even Buerger's disease can be cured with unorthodox treatment

A few years ago, Glen began having trouble with his left leg. He also had angina pectoris. Not only did his chest bother him, but his food and leg also became quite painful. He could walk no more than a block because of the severity of the pain in his leg. His foot was also cold most of the time.

At night Glen would get up and walk about for 15 minutes every so often to relieve the pain. The only way he could sleep was to let his foot hang out of bed. Even then he would wake up every couple of hours.

His doctor diagnosed his problem as Buerger's disease, an ailment in which the person suffers from an inflammation of the inner walls of small blood vessels with constriction and clogging due to blood clots. His doctor told him his condition was incurable since there was no specific therapy available for Buerger's disease.

When Glen came to see me, his foot was a bluish-purple color. He had an ulcer under his big toe. I immediately started him on 2,000 units of vitamin E daily. The first sign of improvement Glen had was a lessening of the pain. Next, the ulcer under his big toe began to heal. His foot lost its bluish-purple color in about eight weeks. It also became warmer, indicating the circulation was better.

Glen has been under my care for a little over a year now. We have seen no sign of the return of his former foot condition. He can now walk long distances without any sign of pain in his leg. Nor does his chest bother him any more. The angina also vanished when he began taking vitamin E. He still takes 1,200 units every day.

How You, Too, Can Keep Your Heart and Circulation Young and Vital

Garlic used to be a standard remedy for high blood pressure, but with the advent of chemotherapy it is considered to be "old-fashioned," especially by medical doctors. However, doctors who still use it have found it to be extremely beneficial in lowering blood pressure without dangerous side effects. Not only have I used it successfully on many of my own patients, but I've used it also on myself. Some years ago my blood pressure was 190 over 110. Today, it is 130 over 85, perfectly normal for a man in his late fifties. I lowered it over a six-month period by using nothing but the garlic therapy, taking from three to five capsules three times a day.

I would far rather use garlic for high blood pressure than reserpine, the medicine most often used in drug therapy. Reserpine's side effects can include drowsiness, nasal stuffiness, gastric distress, bloating, and severe mental depression. The side effects from garlic are better digestion and normalized bowel movements.

It would be wonderful if fat people could lower their blood pressure by garlic alone as Joe did, but to tell the truth, the loss of weight will do much to lower the pressure too, and make you even healthier besides.

The United States Armed Services made a survey of 23,000 men and women to determine the effects of being overweight. This study showed that among men and women of all ages, blood pressure always increased in direct proportion to the amount of excess body fat. The Defense Department also found high blood pressure present two and one half times as often in fat people as in those of normal weight.

When you get rid of your excess fat, your blood pressure will also go down. I know this to be a fact. *I have never seen a single case in all my years of practice where the patient's blood pressure was not lowered as he got rid of his excess fat on my non-glue-food diet.*

Patients who've come to me with blood pressures of 180 to 240 have within a period of six months to a year on my non-glue-food diet lowered those readings to a range of 120 to 150 depending on their ages and the amount of permanent damage in their blood vascular systems. Vitamin E also helps reduce the heart and blood vessel damage.

So if you are fat and have high blood pressure, take it from me. When you reduce, you will lower your blood pressure. It has to work that way since that is nature's way of doing things.

* * *

Minerals can affect your pulse rate. Calcium and magnesium both quiet the pulse. Both are needed for a steady, strong heart beat. A deficiency of potassium can also cause a racing pulse. This happened when the Apollo 15 astronauts suffered a reduction of potassium in their dietary intake. So if you have a rapid pulse rate, 80 or above, take some dolomite and extra potassium. These minerals could solve the problem in short order for you.

* * *

A great many times, the vitamin B complex will solve cases of fibrillation, palpitation, and irregularities of the heart beat. Especially bad for the heart is a deficiency of natural vitamin B-1 or thiamine. This can happen if a person eats too much refined white sugar, for sugar is an *anti-nutrient*. Sugar needs vitamin B for its metabolism, but since it brings none into the body itself, it steals your body's vitamin B reserves and draws them away from areas where they are vitally needed, for example, the heart.

So if you do have irregularities in your heart beat, step up your vitamin B consumption and cut down on your sugar intake. You will be pleasantly surprised at the results.

❀ ❀ ❀

Vitamin E is valuable in treating circulatory conditions, such as varicose veins, hemorrhoids, poor circulation in the hands and feet, phlebitis, Buerger's disease, angina pectoris, and coronary thrombosis. The power of vitamin E to treat or *prevent* all kinds of cardiovascular disease depends upon its four chief characteristics:

1. Vitamin E is a natural anti-thrombin; it keeps clots from forming. It will also dissolve clots that are already formed.

2. It helps conserve oxygen and helps the tissues use oxygen more efficiently.

3. Vitamin E prevents excessive scar tissue production. In many cases, it helps absorb and dissolve unwanted scars.

4. It dilates the blood vessels. It can also open up new pathways in the damaged circulation and bypass blocks caused by clots and hardened arteries.

How to recognize angina pectoris

In angina pectoris the coronary arteries that supply blood to the heart are always on the borderline of insufficiency. There will often be attacks of the same kind of pain as in a true coronary attack of thrombosis. However, with rest the pain will pass without blockage of any of the arteries of the heart.

During an attack of angina, the person will have a gripping pain in the upper chest that often radiates up the left side of the neck and down the left arm. The word angina means *suffocation*. This is often how the patient will describe the attack.

The pain of angina can be brought on by exercise, anxiety or both. The normal drug treatment is a nitroglycerin tablet placed under the tongue. This helps ease the pain and often gives dramatic relief. It does not solve the basic problem, however, which is not enough blood supply to the heart through the coronary arteries.

How vitamin E can help angina pectoris

Vitamin E helps increase the supply of oxygen to all the muscles in the body, especially the heart. Since a lack of oxygen is the problem that triggers the pain of angina, the solution is to supply more oxygen to the heart by increasing the intake of vitamin E.

No other substance has ever been found that works as well as vitamin E in helping the blood get the much needed oxygen to the heart. Remember that nitroglycerin is a drug, not a food. It gives only temporary relief to a person suffering with angina. But vitamin E is a food, not a drug. It helps restore the heart to normal again, not just alleviate the pain temporarily.

I have had many patients once unable to walk even a couple of blocks without suffering anginal pain to recover with vitamin E to the extent they are now able to climb several flights of stairs without any trouble at all.

How to prevent an attack of coronary thrombosis

In a true heart attack where there is a sudden actual blockage or thrombosis of the coronary arteries — as opposed to the temporary insufficiency in the blood supply of angina — the person will have a sudden severe pain in the center of the chest, sometimes radiating across the chest, into the neck or down the arms. The victim will feel a tight crushing sensation and experience a feeling of impending death. He will also suffer from shortness of breath.

The major difference between a coronary heart attack and angina pectoris is the severity of the symptoms. Secondly, since a coronary artery has actually been blocked or occluded in coronary thrombosis, rest will not relieve the attack as in angina.

Immediate emergency treatment in almost every case of coronary thrombosis is imperative if the patient is to live. If the person does survive the attack, several months of convalescence will be needed for the heart to return to a normal state. A full year may be required before he can finally resume his regular normal activities.

If you haven't had this happen to you yet, here's how vitamin E can help you prevent it. First of all, remember vitamin E is a natural anti-coagulant. When you have enough vitamin E in your diet and in your blood stream, you will reduce the chances of having a blood clot forming that could block off your coronary arteries and stop the oxygen supply to your heart. Vitamin E also acts to dilate the blood vessels and open up new pathways in damaged circulation, which will bypass those clogged or hardened blood vessels.

How my heart patients have been helped by vitamin E

Unfortunately, many of my heart patients come to me after the coronary has occurred rather than before. Yet because of vitamin E's ability to act as an anti-coagulant, a clot dissolver and a blood vessel dilator, the oxygen supply to the heart can be increased so the person is able to live a normal, active and happy life again.

Some of my patients are farmers who cannot seem to accept a life without hard work. Nick is one such person. The last time I drove out to his place, he was out in the field helping a neighbor bale hay. He'd already milked and fed six cows, cleaned out the barns, done some other barnyard chores, and it was only 10 o'clock in the morning. Only two years before Nick had been flat on his back in the country hospital with a coronary attack; he was not expected to live. But vitamin E and a proper diet restored his health.

Cliff is another heart patient of mine. He and I go pheasant hunting every fall. That's hard work with a lot of rough walking through the countryside, five to six miles a day. Cliff had a coronary attack five years ago and vitamin E restored him to health too.

As good as vitamin E is, however, it cannot keep your heart and circulation young and vital by itself alone. If you smoke, if you get too little exercise or if you're overweight, then don't expect vitamin E to solve all these problems for you too. If you want to avoid that heart attack and add many active and vigorous, happy years to your life, you'll have to do something about those problems as well.

How mild exercise can help your heart

Remember I told you that muscular activity helps bring the blood back to the heart from the extremities, the hands and feet? That's one of the main reasons mild exercise like walking is good for you. It reduces the load on your heart. When you walk, don't just stroll. Go at a good brisk clip. But don't jog or run. Walk fast. Running and jogging, unless you're in top physical condition, can stop your heart just as quickly and surely as playing tennis or shoveling snow.

Not that I'm against playing tennis — I'm not. But I recommend that you don't go at it the way so many businessmen do, trying to be weekend athletes. Ease into it gradually so your heart can adjust itself to the new work loads. You can't slop around until you're 50 or 60 and expect to gain back the physique you had when you were 20 in a week.

Sudden, violent exercise when you're not used to it, like tennis or shoveling snow, can damage your heart by overloading it. When I lived in Missouri, I never shoveled snow off my driveway. I figured the weatherman put it there and he could take it away. He never failed me: sooner or later, all that snow disappeared without one bit of help from me.

12

How to Quickly and Easily Correct Your Low Blood Sugar with Drugless Dietary Methods

Do you suffer from depression, insomnia, anxiety, irritability, inability to concentrate, crying spells, forgetfulness, confusion, anti-social behavior? Do you often have headaches, dizziness, trembling, numbness, blurred vision, staggering, fainting or blackouts, muscular twitching? Are you troubled with exhaustion, fatigue, bloating, abdominal cramps, muscle and joint pains, stomach cramps, colitis? Have you gone to your doctor time after time looking for help only to be told, "There's nothing actually wrong with you...it's all in your mind...you're a bit neurotic...you'll have to learn to live with it"?

Well, I can assure you there's definitely something wrong if you have any of these symptoms. Chances are you have low blood sugar. *One in every ten persons has.* In fact, without even seeing you or talking with you, I can tell you this: *if you have at least three of the following symptoms, it's almost a cinch you have hypoglycemia.*

1. Chronic fatigue
2. Chronic nervous exhaustion
3. Afternoon headaches
4. Eat often, get hunger pangs, or feel faint
5. Feel weak and faint if meals are delayed
6. Fatigue that is relieved by eating
7. Get shaky and weak when hungry
8. Sleepy after meals

   9. Sleep during the day

10. Lack of energy

11. Often depressed

Don't blame your doctor altogether for not diagnosing your ailment properly. After all, he's only following the example set for him. You see, back in 1973 the American Medical Association said hypoglycemia was a "nondisease." So if hypoglycemia is not a *real* illness, how could your doctor diagnose your condition? In spite of such silly nonsense, both you and I know hypoglycemia is for real. I know something else, too — you don't have to live with it. You can correct it with the proper foods and specific vitamins I'll tell you about in this chapter.

It is important to get rid of low blood sugar. It in itself is bad enough, but *it is only a forerunner of far worse things to come.* It is only the beginning of other chronic and degenerative conditions that will bother you as you get older — heart disease, hypertension, digestive ailments, skin conditions, rheumatism, arthritis, and the like, *depending upon which part of your body is the weakest.* I will cover a few of these conditions here so you can get an idea of all the troubles low blood sugar can eventually cause for you. Right now, let me give you an example of a typical case of hypoglycemia.

How low blood sugar can sap your strength and drain your energy

"Why am I so darned worn out all the time, Doc?" a patient asked me the other day. "I just don't seem to have enough energy to get my work done at all. I drag around the office all day long."

"I can best explain that to you by discussing your daily food intake, Homer," I responded. "For instance, you've already told me that all you have for breakfast is a cup of black coffee and a cigarette. Homer, when you don't eat enough, when you miss a meal or when you eat the wrong kind of food, your blood sugar falls, causing all those symptoms you already know only too well.

"Of course, your coffee and cigarette give you a temporary

lift, but it doesn't last; so soon you become tense, irritable and overly tired. You get a headache. You feel miserable all over and your body develops an insatiable craving for something sweet. So you'll overeat at the next meal, or you'll probably stuff yourself even before then at your mid-morning coffee break with such man-made carbohydrates as doughnuts, sweet rolls, pastry, pie, cake or some other sweet.

"Your body then absorbs more sugar into the blood stream than it needs to meet your immediate energy requirements. Your blood sugar rises above normal limits so your body reacts at once to get rid of your *hyper*glycemia. Your pancreas is stimulated to produce insulin so the excess sugar in your blood can be removed. Otherwise, the excess sugar in your blood would spill over into your urine as in diabetes.

"But the trouble is, Homer, your pancreas is overactive as a result of the constant input of sugar into your blood stream from all the man-made carbohydrates you're always eating. Not only does your pancreas remove the excess sugar from your blood, but *it also removes more than it should,* so your blood sugar immediately falls below normal limits shortly after you've eaten. Again, you experience symptoms of hypoglycemia: tension, irritability, headache, excessive fatigue, nausea, and an insatiable desire for sweets.

"What do you do then, Homer? Well, if it's lunch time, you'll load yourself down with man-made carbohydrates again: white bread, rolls, spaghetti, pizza, cake, pie a la mode, and so on. You leave no room at all for the high energy proteins and natural carbohydrate foods your body needs so much. If it's mid-afternoon, you'll grab a couple of doughnuts or a sweet roll, maybe a piece of cake with ice cream for your coffee break. You might even take a candy bar or two back to your desk. And that same vicious cycle repeats itself all over again.

"You see, the more sugary foods you eat, the hungrier you become, and the more tired and worn out you feel. You go home from the office each day absolutely exhausted even when you didn't get any work done, and you can't understand why you're always so tired and worn out.

"Your natural tendency is to blame the way you feel on the

fast pace of earning a living or the intense pressure of these modern times. To tell the truth, Homer, the way you feel is a result of eating all those man-made carbohydrates — those packaged, canned and processed artificial foods that are loaded down with sugar. Replace them with high animal proteins such as beef, lamb, poultry, fish, milk, eggs and cheese. Eat lots of fresh fruits and vegetables; they'll give you all the carbohydrates you need. Use stone-ground 100 percent whole wheat bread and whole grain cereals. When you do this, Homer, you'll feel like a million every day. You'll have all the energy you need."

And that's what happened. When Homer followed my advice, his hypoglycemia with all its symptoms of fatigue and exhaustion vanished.

What actually happens in your body when you have low blood sugar

I'm sure you can see from Homer's example that a high sugar intake causes low blood sugar. This seems like a physiological paradox, but I know any lingering doubts in your mind will be cleared up when you finish reading this short section.

You see, the normal body keeps its blood sugar at a quite constant level. But when a person's carbohydrate metabolism is not working properly, when it has been damaged or thrown out of kilter by the constant and excessive consumption of man-made carbohydrates, then the blood sugar fluctuates up and down abnormally. The ingested sugar is absorbed so rapidly into the blood stream that the blood sugar rises far above its normal limits.

Under normal circumstances, the pancreas would secrete just enough insulin to bring the blood sugar down to its proper level. Unfortunately, over a period of time due to the constant and heavy consumption of man-made foods containing refined white sugar and bleached white flour — for example, white bread, rolls, doughnuts, cake, cookies, ice cream, candy, soft drinks, etc. the pancreas actually becomes trigger-happy. It secretes far too much insulin at the slightest hint of excess sugar in the blood.

When too much insulin enters the blood stream at one time, the blood sugar falls rapidly below normal limits. A person with hypoglycemia will experience a wide range of symptoms which I've already mentioned. Too often people with hypoglycemia think more sugar is the answer since they usually feel better, *but only temporarily,* after eating sweets, drinking coffee, consuming alcohol or smoking cigarettes. But that is not true. The only cure for low blood sugar and its associated ailments is not more sugar, but less sugar in the diet.

How Ralph quickly conquered his low blood sugar with these unusually easy-to-use methods

A little over a year ago, Ralph was hospitalized for a nervous breakdown. He had fallen into a deep depression. He lost all ambition, became extremely nervous and was unable to do his job properly. He could not relax or sleep at night.

Despite a variety of tests and a complete physical examination, Ralph was released from the hospital without a positive diagnosis as to what his problem was. In fact, his doctor told him he could find nothing wrong with him at all. He told Ralph to take a vacation, change his job or develop a hobby — that sort of vague, abstract advice.

Completely discouraged by all this, Ralph came to me for help. As soon as he told me his symptoms, I suspected low blood sugar and a vitamin B deficiency. My analysis of his dietary intake along with some other diagnostic laboratory tests confirmed my suspicions.

I immediately asked Ralph to stop using refined white sugar and to avoid all compound man-made foods containing it. I asked him to get plenty of animal protein in his diet and to eat fresh fruits and vegetables, as well as 100 percent whole wheat bread and natural whole grain cereals. I also had Ralph take a high potency vitamin B supplement (B-50) three times a day, along with some dessicated liver and yeast.

After only a few weeks on his new dietary regime for low blood sugar, Ralph felt like a brand new person. He no longer was troubled with any of his previous symptoms. In fact, getting rid of his hypoglycemia helped Ralph to get a promotion. The last time he was in to see me, Ralph said his boss had been on the verge of firing him when he went to the hospital, but his work had improved so much after he'd been to me that he'd been promoted instead.

What refined white sugar can do to babies and children

I have found that a great many skin rashes, various kinds of allergies, infections, catarrhal conditions with excessive phlegm, upset stomachs, as well as nervous problems in babies will improve just as soon as refined white sugar or syrup is taken out of their formulas.

In 95 out of 100 cases when a mother brings an undernourished child to me, I find that the child is underweight and suffering from malnutrition due to the excessive consumption of products containing sugar and syrup, as well as the absence of body-building proteins. Such foods eaten either during or between meals will destroy the appetite completely for healthy and nourishing natural foods like fresh fruits and vegetables, which are so necessary for normal growth.

I also find that these children have almost always been given cake, candy, ice cream and so on as a reward for eating only a small amount of vegetables or drinking just a little bit of milk. This is a mistake, for sugar is habit forming, just like alcohol or tobacco. The child will develop a desire for sweet man-made carbohydrates that will be hard to break in later life. Excessive sugar consumption will also interfere with the absorption and metabolism of calcium which is so necessary for the proper formation of bones and teeth in the growing child. Calcium is also needed for proper heart action and blood coagulation.

How Eddie overcame his lack of energy and regained his health

More than once I have treated children in my practice who, although not suffering from a gross form of protein malnutrition, have presented a variety of vague symptoms that their previous doctors had dismissed as imaginary or unimportant.

Just for instance, there was Eddie, a ten-year-old fifth-grader. Eddie lacked energy, his mother told me; he had no desire to play outdoors with his friends. She said he was lazy, always sleepy, dragged around the house, and seemed listless and completely indifferent to what was going on around him. His school grades were poor. He brought home mostly D's with an occasional C, even though his aptitude tests indicated he had a high IQ and a good learning potential.

My physical examination showed Eddie was several pounds underweight and most definitely anemic. A thorough questioning of his dietary habits revealed that he consumed a tremendous amount of sugar. His mother had read an advertisement saying sugar was the best source of quick energy so she forced sweets on Eddie constantly, hoping they would snap him out of his lethargy — but they only made him worse. Eddie was also extremely deficient in vitamin B.

I placed Eddie on my diet for low blood sugar with explicit instructions not to eat any sugar at all, either by itself or in any compound food or drink. I also gave him a high potency vitamin B supplement (B-50) to be taken twice a day, morning and noon, along with some dessicated liver and yeast tablets to be taken three times a day.

Eddie and his mother cooperated willingly and in only a few short weeks he changed completely. He was full of pep and energy and seemed never to tire out. In two months he was up to his normal weight, and his anemia disappeared too. Even his next report card was most gratifying to see, for it carried evidence of the change that had taken place: Eddie brought home two A's, three B's, only one C, and not a single D or F.

Effects of sugar on the body in middle and old age

In middle and old age, any number of chronic degenerative conditions can result from the excessive consumption of sugar. For example, eating too much sugar is often a predisposing cause of arthritis, neuritis and rheumatism, as well as many other chronic diseases.

Indigestion with gas on the stomach and bowel is a common ailment of middle aged and elderly people. Sugar irritates the mucous membranes of the digestive tract and causes increased muscular tension of the stomach and bowel. The abnormal tightness and muscular contraction of the digestive system causes a constriction of the food passages which delays the emptying time of the stomach. When food is held back, the sugar ferments. This forms gas, causing cramps, pain and many other symptoms of indigestion that are some of the signs of hypoglycemia.

How Eileen got rid of her digestive problems

I have no idea how many patients come to me suffering from indigestion of some sort just from eating too much sugar. Eileen was one. Her stomach cramps were so severe they would completely double her over in pain. After only one week on my diet for hypoglycemia along with a vitamin B supplement and without any sugar whatever, her cramps and gas pains stopped. That was more than a year ago, and her problem has never returned.

Other ailments caused by refined white sugar

Refined white sugar will lower the hydrochloric acid content of the stomach. A low gastric acidity is extremely common in middle-aged and elderly people suffering from hypoglycemia. This lowered stomach acidity is often confused with acid stomach or heartburn. The person then takes an alkaline medication to neutralize the acid and relieve the pain when actually the real trouble is not enough acid in the stomach in the first place.

Although the person may get some temporary relief from this medication, the condition will only continue to get worse. These alkaline anti-acids that you can buy over the counter without a prescription have never cured a stomach condition and they never will, for they treat only the symptoms and do not eliminate the basic cause of the condition. Not only that, they are dangerous in that they can cause osteomalacia as I mentioned back in Chapter 6 on page 99.

My own father took baking soda for years and years for his heartburn and never got any better. I can remember seeing him head for the kitchen cupboard after every meal to reach for the baking soda. One day I got him to try a couple of spoonfuls of vinegar in a glass of water *with* his meal, and to his amazement, he got up from the table without heartburn for the first time in 20 years or more. He never returned to the baking soda again; as long as he used a bit of vinegar in a glass of water *with* his meals, he never had to.

How Norman got rid of his sour stomach without dangerous alkalizers

When Norman came to see me, he was taking anti-acids after every meal and between meals besides. In the beginning, just like my father, he had used baking soda but he eventually furned to the commercial over-the-counter alkaline medications you see advertised on TV all the time. These gave him temporary relief, but he finally got tired of taking them and decided to see if I could help his condition.

I know sometimes the treatment I use for hypoglycemia is so simple that it's hard for people to believe it works, but all I did was have Norman stop eating sugar in all its forms, go on my basic diet for hypoglycemia, and take some vitamin B along with dessicated liver and yeast tablets. I didn't have to tell Normal to stop taking his anti-acid medications. Within a week he had no need for any of them. He has never used them again. How long ago was that? More years than I care to count.

This low stomach acidity, which comes from the overuse of refined white sugar and is one of the main symptoms of hypoglycemia, will often lead to other chronic and degenerative diseases seen especially in older patients. For instance, when the stomach acidity is too low, iron is not readily absorbed from the food. As a result, it is hard for the body to make up its iron losses (this is particularly true in women) and the person then suffers from anemia.

How Helen cured her anemia in short order

Helen was suffering from anemia. She had been taking an iron supplement (which is the usual treatment most doctors use) for several months with only slight improvement. She became dissatisfied with her progress and came to me. I found she had a low gastric acidity along with hypoglycemia, so I had her eliminate all refined white sugar from her diet and put her on my diet for low blood sugar along with vitamin B, liver and yeast tablets.

I continued an iron supplement for her anemia, and this time it was effective: as soon as the sugar was removed from her dietary intake and vitamin B supplements were added, her stomach acidity increased and the iron was then easily absorbed and assimilated by her body. In only a month her blood tests were back to normal and she was feeling like a million.

How Clyde recovered from his heart attack with this exceptional method

Patients who have come to me with all the signs and symptoms of coronary heart disease have lost those symptoms in just a few short months by eliminating sugar in all its forms and adding vitamins B and E to their diets. One such person who comes to mind is Clyde. He suffered a heart attack while on vacation in Minnesota. After several months in the hospital he returned home, classified as completely disabled for social security benefits. He continued to suffer periodic chest pains and pain radiating down the inside of his left arm, with concurrent fainting spells and heavy sweating.

My dietary diagnosis of Clyde's food intake revealed a heavy sugar intake. I placed him on my basic diet for hypoglycemia along with a vitamin B supplement (B-50 twice a day) and some dessicated liver and yeast tablets. I also gave him 1,200 units of vitamin E each day to help repair his heart damage and restore its normal function again.

Three months after Clyde first came to see me, his symptoms began to lessen. They became less frequent and not as severe as before. At the end of six months, they became almost nonexistent. Clyde has not suffered an attack of any sort for more than two years.

He lives a completely normal life now. He takes a walk each day for a couple of miles, plays 18 holes of golf each week, and bowls in a senior citizen's league. Clyde is enjoying his retirement completely and has forgotten all about his heart attack.

Why refined white sugar is not a "real" food

A food is properly defined as any substance that serves to nourish and build up or replace and repair the tissues when it is taken into the body. A food will sustain life and promote growth. Refined white sugar will do none of these. It cannot be used to build vital muscle tissue, blood or bone. Sugar cannot be used to replace and repair body tissues; it will not support life, nor will it encourage growth. In fact, just the opposite is true. In experiments conducted at Washington University's School of Medicine, it was found that when sugar was fed to rats, it stopped their normal growth and greatly shortened their life expectancy.

Sugar can be stored in warehouses for years and years without spoiling. *Any food that will not spoil is not worth eating.* In fact, if it will not spoil, it is not fit to eat. Only foods that have nutritive value — protein, fats, natural carbohydrates, vitamins, minerals, and enzymes — will deteriorate and spoil.

Refined white sugar does not have a single vitamin, mineral or enzyme in it. Every single nutritive element initially found in it has been removed. The original food, sugar beets or sugar cane, has been reduced to the level of an organic chemical that contains calories but has no food value of any sort. In fact, it is an anti-nutrient, a starvation food, as you'll see right now...

Why refined white sugar is a starvation food

Sugar is called a starvation food because it steals your body's vitamin B reserves and draws them away from areas where they are vitally needed. Large quantities of vitamin B, especially thiamine, are necessary for the absorption and assimilation of sugar. Since sugar has no vitamins of any sort, the body has no choice but to draw upon its own vitamin B reserves to metabolize the sugar. The more sugar you consume, the more vitamin B is stolen from your body. This is bad for the heart, which uses large quantities of vitamin B, especially thiamine, to function properly. The shortage of vitamin B in the body can also contribute to emotional instability.

How much sugar do you think you eat?

Many of my patients find it hard to believe that they eat too much sugar until I give them some basic facts about the average diet. Take Tom, for instance:

"Doc, I never use sugar in my coffee," Tom said. "And I seldom eat cereal so I don't use much sugar there. In fact, I can't recall when I've used a single spoon of sugar in anything. I don't see how it could be causing my problems."

"Tom, you eat sugar and you don't even know it," I said. "Tell me, do you ever eat glazed doughnuts? Seems to me I've seen you in the Mister Donut place at one time or another."

"Yes, Doc, I do," Tom said. "I always stop there on my way to the office and have two glazed doughnuts and coffee every morning."

"You take in 12 teaspoons of sugar every time you do that, Tom," I said. "Each glazed doughnut contains at least six teaspoons of sugar. And tell me, Tom. Do you ever eat cake? Cupcakes? Use jelly on your toast? Syrup on your pancakes? Eat pie or ice cream? How about a candy bar now and then? Ever drink a coke or a root beer?"

"Sure," Tom said. "But I don't use sugar as such and that's what we're talking about, isn't it?"

"Tom, you use sugar and you don't even realize it," I said. "For instance, a piece of angel food cake has seven teaspoons of sugar. A little cupcake with frosting has six; a chocolate eclair, seven. A teaspoon of grape jelly for your toast has the concentrated equivalent of five teaspoons of sugar; strawberry jam, four. A twelve-ounce bottle of the average soft drink has from six to ten teaspoons of sugar. A piece of pie contains at least eleven and a candy bar, seven. So you see, Tom, you take in a lot of sugar each day even though you may never reach for the sugar bowl itself."

I'm sure you, too, just like Tom, consume sugar all day long even if you never go near the sugar bowl either. It's always there in all those man-made packaged and processed carbohydrate foods. Read the label carefully and you'll see.

Refined white sugar: a summary

1. Refined white sugar is not a "real" food. It has no vitamins, minerals, enzymes, proteins, fats or natural carbohydrates. It furnishes only calories to the body. It has no nutrients that will sustain life and promote growth. It cannot be used to build vital muscle tissue, blood or bone. It is the basic cause of hypoglycemia.

2. Refined white sugar is an anti-nutrient, a starvation food. Vitamin and mineral deficiencies result from its use. Instead of furnishing vitamins to the body, it draws them from your body reserves for its metabolism, thus depleting especially the vitamin B complex.

3. You can get all the energy you need from the natural carbohydrates in fresh fruits and vegetables. Other wholesome foods like dairy products, meat, fish, eggs, honey, and unprocessed whole grains furnish plenty of calories for your body's daily energy requirements.

4. Just like alcohol and tobacco, sugar is habit forming. It is found in almost all of today's packaged, canned and modern processed foods. The best way to avoid sugar is to eat primarily fresh fruits and fresh vegetables. Eat foods that are grown, not foods that are made.

5. Sugar is responsible for many of the chronic and degenerative diseases of middle and old age, as well as the ailments of babies and children. Sugar consumption can result not only in hypoglycemia, but also in tooth decay, diabetes, indigestion, gas, constipation, skin diseases, anemia, excess weight, infections, colds, and sinusitis. It is also a contributing factor in bronchitis, arthritis, rheumatism, neuritis, coronary heart disease, lowered physical efficiency, chronic fatigue and headaches.

6. If you will avoid eating refined white sugar and the

foods in which it is found, you can expect to live a much healthier and longer life with greater freedom from those chronic diseases and complaints that trouble most people in middle and old age.

How You Can Keep from Getting
Low Blood Sugar Yourself

First of all, eliminate all refined white sugar and man-made carbohydrates from your daily diet. Read the labels on all canned and packaged foods to see if sugar has been added — 99 times out of 100 it has. *You do not need one ounce of refined white sugar to provide your body with energy.* Don't let the sugar industry's advertising mislead you. Natural carbohydrates in fresh fruits and vegetables will furnish all the energy your body needs. You can always use honey as a natural sweetener. But be wise: although honey is a natural sugar with vitamins, minerals, and enzymes, you should use it sparingly if you are prone to have low blood sugar.

* * *

Eat plenty of animal protein in the form of fresh meat, fish, poultry, milk, eggs and cheese. Avoid meats that have been processed with sodium nitrate and sodium nitrite. These are potent cancer-causing chemicals. Bacon is considered by many scientists to be the most dangerous food in the supermarket. Eat plenty of fresh fruits and vegetables, raw if possible. These will give you natural carbohydrates, vitamins, minerals, enzymes, cellulose, fiber and energy. Use stone-ground 100 percent whole wheat bread and whole grain cereals.

* * *

Take a high potency vitamin B supplement such as the B-50 or B-100 twice a day (morning and noon), along with some dessicated liver and yeast tablets three times a day. Large doses of vitamin B, especially niacin and pyridoxine help to stabilize your blood sugar levels. Both B-50 and B-100 have ample quantities of these two vitamins of the B complex. If you are troubled by excessive fatigue, take a wheat germ oil supplement at mealtime, too.

13

How to Solve or Prevent
the Special Problems of Older Age
Easily, Safely and Painlessly

First off, let me say that this chapter will not cover all the problems you might feel are identified with older age. I have already covered many of them in preceding chapters, for instance, arthritis, rheumatism, cardiovascular conditions, and certain digestive problems. This is not to say that these ailments afflict only those who are older. They can happen to anyone at any age, but they most often occur in people who are in their fifties and above.

So if you are in your twenties, thirties, or even your forties, you might think this chapter will not benefit you. If that's what you're thinking, I must tell you that you're wrong. Here's why...

An extremely exhaustive and detailed study made by a large insurance company shows that by the time people reach the age of 45, two out of every three have some sort of chronic diseased condition. By the time they are 65, that figure has jumped to eight out of every ten.

But the seeds of these degenerative diseases have been sown much, much earlier than the age of 45. By the time the average person reaches his early or mid-thirties, he wonders what has happened to the zip and zest he used to have for living back in his teens and twenties.

Actually, chronic and degenerative diseases are already beginning to take their toll when a person is barely into his thirties — the effects just don't show up for a long time. Usually, the symptoms are just too vague to permit the average doctor to tag the condition with a specific name. What has caused these chronic ailments to start? Bacteria or viruses as in the child-hood diseases of mumps, measles, chicken pox? No indeed. They have started due to inadequate diet and improper nutri-tion. I have confirmed that fact over and over again by the clinical results I've obtained in case after case by using vita-mins, minerals, and the proper diet of natural foods to cure the patient's disease.

When you read the case histories in this chapter and see how people have resolved their problems, it will no doubt oc-cur to you that if a certain vitamin or mineral can cure a con-dition, then using that vitamin or mineral before you have the ailment will prevent it. If that's the way you feel after reading this book, I will have accomplished my purpose. You'll be on your way to better health.

How Adrian keeps his "old" bones strong and healthy

Adrian has been a patient of mine for many years now. His original complaint, a duodenal ulcer, was resolved many years ago, but he has continued to come to my office every month for a check-up. He has taken natural vitamins and minerals and avoided white sugar and white flour since he first started com-ing to me for treatment.

Shortly after Adrian's 84th birthday, he fell from a step ladder while putting up a storm window. He fell about five feet down hard on his cement driveway, but he did not suffer any broken bones. He had a big bump on his right thigh, a little soreness in his right ankle, and a skinned right elbow.

Adrian's neighbor saw him fall and came to help him up, thinking he had perhaps broken his hip. But he had not, thanks to the 4,000 milligrams of calcium he was getting each day from the dolomite I had asked him to take. Adrain told me he didn't even feel any stiffness or lameness the next day after his fall in his hip although he had fallen squarely on it.

How Beatrice keeps her fingernails firm and strong

Beatrice came to me to see if I could do anything to help her strengthen her fingernails. They were so thin and weak that they were almost like tissue paper. They broke very easily and she was constantly snagging them. My dietary analysis revealed that Beatrice was terribly deficient in her calcium intake. I gave her 5,000 milligrams of calcium each day in the form of dolomite. At the end of only ten days Beatrice's nails were becoming stronger and thicker. At the end of three weeks, they were completely normal.

The calcium also strengthened Beatrice's entire bone structure. Several years before she came to see me, Beatrice had slipped on an icy sidewalk, fallen and broken her hip. At that time she was not taking any calcium at all, so her bones were fragile and weak.

But that is not true any more. Last week Beatrice fell down a flight of stairs after tripping over a small rug at the top. Her X-rays showed no broken bones at all, which is amazing since Beatrice is 76. Such a fall could easily have broken some bones in a much younger person; but she had only a few bruises and sore spots here and there, thanks to dolomite.

How Olivia marvelously solved one of the special problems of older age

Olivia came to me seeking help for nervous exhaustion. She was 63 years old. My dietary diagnosis revealed that she was extremely deficient in calcium, magnesium and pyridoxine (vitamin B-6). Olivia told me the doctor had removed eight kidney stones in an operation a few years ago. He placed her on a diet that restricted her calcium intake, saying this would prevent further kidney stone formation. But in spite of this calcium-poor diet, she passed stones at various times after her operation. These were extremely painful ordeals for her. To top it off, her low calcium diet had made her a nervous wreck. So she came to me for help.

I asked Olivia to take 150 milligrams of pyridoxine each day. I also had her take a high potency vitamin B supplement (B-50) three times a day so she would have a balanced vitamin B intake. Three capsules of B-50 have 150 milligrams of pydoxine so Olivia was getting 300 milligrams a day of B-6. I gave her magnesium tablets as well as dolomite for her calcium and magnesium shortage. Here's why these supplements were needed in her case.

Kidney stones are primarily calcium oxalate. Magnesium helps hold the oxalic acid in solution in the urine, preventing it from precipitating out as oxalate particles that can eventually clump together with calcium to form kidney stones.

Vitamin B-6 helps control the body's production of oxalic acid, thus limiting the amount that reaches the kidneys. I also asked Olivia to avoid foods that are high in oxalic acid: chocolate, cocoa, tea, rhubarb, spinach, chard, parsley, and beet tops. I also told her to avoid asparagus, which can aggravate existing kidney complaints.

Even though kidney stones are most often composed of calcium oxalate, I had Olivia take some dolomite, which also contains magnesium, and eat plenty of calcium-rich foods since her body was so calcium starved. As long as she was getting the magnesium and pyridoxine she needed to keep minerals in solution in the urine, the amount of calcium in her diet would not be a contributing factor in the formation of kidney stones. A person simply cannot go without calcium and remain in good health. Calcium is an absolute must in nutrition and of course, in Olivia's case, her calcium deficiency had caused her nervous exhaustion and cardiac palpitations.

Now what have been the results? Olivia has been my patient now for nearly five years. Her extreme nervousness disappeared within a month after she came to see me. Regular kidney checks have shown absolutely no sign of stone formation. Olivia now leads a happy, healthy, normal and active life. She has more pep and energy than lots of people I've seen in their fifties although she is now nearing 70.

Lee's prostate problem quickly responds to fantastic treatment

I have dozens of case histories that show how prostate problems can be quickly relieved by this extraordinary method. Lee's case is a typical example.

A few years ago Lee, who was then 67, began to suffer with all the usual symptoms of an enlarged prostate gland. He had a continual desire to urinate, yet he could pass only a small amount of urine at a time. The stream was also much smaller than normal. Lee suffered a great deal of pain and discomfort during urination. His bladder seemed full all the time and he was constantly aware of a dull ache across the lower part of his abdomen. Lee's condition also greatly disturbed his sleep. He would get up five or six times a night to go to the bathroom, only to find he could dribble only a few drops.

At that time, the doctor he was seeing advised surgery to resolve his condition, but Lee was not ready for such a drastic procedure. Instead, he came to me to see if I could help him avoid an operation. My dietary analysis revealed that Lee was extremely deficient in zinc. I was not surprised to find this, for a zinc deficiency exists in almost every case of an enlarged prostate.

I placed Lee on 30 milligrams of zinc each day along with six bee pollen tablets, a supplemental measure I have always found to be valuable in prostate problems. I asked him to take these supplements in equal amounts with each meal. Within only a month, Lee's condition began to improve. It continued to do so and at the end of six months, Lee said he felt completely well again. He could urinate without any discomfort whatever. He slept all night without getting up unless he drank too much water or milk before going to bed. Even then he got up no more than once.

A year after he first came to me, Lee was examined by the same doctor who had recommended an operation and was told he had no more prostate trouble to worry about. The doctor just couldn't understand what had happened to clear up Lee's condition.

How Charlotte prevents the skin problems of older age

Charlotte is 77 years old, and she is in excellent health. Her face doesn't have a single wrinkle in it; her skin is smooth, soft, and beautiful. How does she do it? Well, she doesn't smoke, doesn't get too much sun on her face, she avoids white sugar and white flour and takes all the vitamins and minerals I recommend. She also does two more things on her own which she says add the finishing touches to give her a perfect complexion.

For years now Charlotte has been using a brewer's yeast face mask and vitamin E skin cream each night before going to bed. She mixes some powdered brewer's yeast in water and applies the mixture to her face. She allows this to dry and leaves it on for about ten minutes. Then she washes it off and applies a vitamin E vanishing cream to her face massaging it in. Charlotte says the brewer's yeast cleanses her pores and tightens her skin while the vitamin E skin cream helps to keep her complexion soft, smooth, and supple. I certainly cannot disagree with what she says — her face is radiantly young. It is living proof that what she's doing is the right thing for her to do.

How to keep your sex life vigorously alive when you're older

Sexual problems do not normally bring older patients to my office; they come for other reasons. However, in the process of taking their case histories, I often find that many of them have given up sexual relations with their partners assuming they're just "over the hill" and nothing can be done about it.

Take Gale, for instance. He was in his early sixties. He told me he had sexual intercourse with his wife only once a month, if then. She was perfectly willing and physically able, but he had simply been unable to maintain an erection hard enough to make love to her. Gale said his wife was sympathetic and understanding, but he knew she was frustrated and wished he were sexually more capable.

Gale's dietary analysis revealed a lack of vitamin F, a deficiency I often find in older men who are impotent and incapable of satisfactory sexual intercourse. Actually, the essential fatty acids are not vitamins in the strictest sense since they are required by the human body in *grams* rather than milligrams for good health.

The essential fatty acids, or vitamin F, are absolutely essential for a normal healthy sex drive. They are found in sunflower, safflower, corn, cottonseed, soybean and peanut oils. They are *not* found in olive oil. I had Gale take two tablespoons of sunflower oil (my favorite) each day, one tablespoon at breakfast, the other with supper. Within less than a month, he was enjoying normal sexual relations with his wife at least once a week, sometimes more often.

How Jim amazingly extended his prime of life

Jim came to me for a vascular problem (venous thrombosis) more than five years ago. Even though I cleared up his condition in less than two months, he has continued to take 1,200 units of vitamin E each day all this time as a preventive measure to prevent any further cardiovascular conditions from developing.

Jim recently applied for some additional life insurance. His agent, who is a friend but not a patient of mine, called me the other day and said, "Doc, what in the world are you doing for Jim T., anyway? He looks to be in better health than he was when he first came to me for insurance more than ten years ago. I swear he doesn't look as if he's aged a bit. Not a wrinkle anywhere. Did he discover the fountain of youth in your office? Let me in on your secret, Doc. Whatever it is you're doing for Jim, I want you to do it for me, too."

"Forrest, it's the vitamin E," I said. "It'll add at least eight years or more to your prime of life for you. Come see me. I can do the same thing for you that I've done for Jim."

How Henry recovered his health completely after the age of 62

I especially want to tell you about Henry. He is living proof of what the proper diet, along with the correct vitamin and mineral supplements, can do for you.

Several years ago when Henry was just 62 years old, his hair was completely white. He was bothered with arthritis and rheumatism in both shoulders and had been hospitalized for several months with a heart attack. Henry's doctor told him he should quit his job, retire early, and take it easy if he wanted to live for a few more years. But Henry felt he couldn't afford to do that. He wanted to wait until he was 65 so he could draw full benefits from his company pension plan and social security, so he went back to work again.

But things went from bad to worse. Henry developed a lingering ankle infection as a result of an accident in the plant. His doctor was hesitant to operate because of Henry's heart condition and the possibility of a thrombosis. Antibiotics had no effect on the ankle infection and Henry's strength slowly drained away because of it. At last he had no choice left: he was forced to retire.

After sitting around for a year in a rocking chair feeling sorry for himself, Henry was almost physically helpless. A few minutes of work of any sort or a little bit of exercise left him deathly sick and fatigued. Finally, in desperation Henry threw all his medicines down the drain and came to see me.

My dietary analysis of Henry's food intake revealed that he was deficient in every single vitamin and mineral. And no wonder. He was living on nothing but man-made carbohydrates — packaged and processed junk foods utterly devoid of natural vitamins and minerals.

I gave him a high potency multi-vitamin, multi-mineral supplement as a base and then added vitamins and minerals individually until he was taking far in excess of the amounts recommended by the Federal Food and Drug Administration as the minimum daily allowances. I'll have more to say about that in the next chapter.

I asked Henry to completely avoid white sugar, white flour and all the products made with them. He was to eat only fresh fruits and vegetables, stone-ground 100 percent whole wheat bread and whole grain cereals along with fresh meat (not canned or preserved), fish, poultry, milk, eggs and cheese for a high-protein intake. I asked Henry to use only unsaturated vegetable fats and oils. To help his ankle infection I used a vitamin E ointment in addition to his vitamin E that he took orally. Of course, the vitamin E helped his heart condition, too.

The results, after only two years of the proper natural foods, vitamins, and minerals without drugs or medicines of any sort, are little short of amazing: Henry's ankle infection healed completely in less than six months; and he no longer suffers the pains of arthritis or rheumatism in his shoulders, nor does he have any sign of heart trouble.

He says his strength and energy are back to where they were when he was in his forties. Henry plays 18 holes of golf every week. He also swims at the YMCA at least twice a week. He enjoys a healthy, happy, vigorous and active life. And the most amazing thing of all is this: Henry's hair, which used to be pure white, is now turning brown again, evidently as a result of the high amount of PABA (Paraminobenzoic acid) in his vitamin B supplement.

How the proper physical activity can keep you young and prevent the special problems of older age

Spokesmen for the department of physical education at a large midwestern university say that studies of men, who are athletic in their youth and continue their physical activities throughout their life show that many of the symptoms of aging can be postponed by as much as ten to fifteen years. In fact, the studies show that men who are physically active will remain in their prime of life even up through their sixties and early or mid-seventies.

One university professor says there is no question in his mind that regular exercise of the correct intensity and duration can postpone the physical deterioration that often occurs as a person grows older.

Now the right kind of exercise can keep you young and prevent many of the special problems of older age — I agree with that. But the wrong kind of physical activity can also kill you. Let me tell you about the wrong kind first.

I once had a neighbor (not a patient of mine) who did not want to lose weight by dieting. Otto liked to eat too much. He wanted to get rid of his excess fat by exercise, specifically running.

Otto was 56 years old and weighed nearly 225 pounds; his blood pressure was also high. He bought a heavy sweat suit and set a route through the neighborhood of three miles.

Every afternoon when he got home from work, on went the sweat suit and out went Otto to run his route. He would come home drenched with perspiration, completely exhausted. Then he would sit down to recover his strength by loading up with man-made carbohydrates: beer, pretzels, potato chips, sandwiches. After he rested for a while, he would eat supper.

He lost about five or six pounds — mostly water — that way in a month. He was unhappy with the results and lengthened his route to four miles. I tried to persuade Otto to stop his running and told him he was going to kill himself if he kept it up, that some day his heart wouldn't take such strenuous exercise any longer and that it would stop on him. But he didn't agree with me. I went to his funeral last summer.

Now for the right kind. Personally, I like to take long walks at a brisk pace. Walking strengthens your leg and thigh muscles. It helps your varicose veins, speeds up your circulation and strengthens your heart. Walking also helps your digestion, elimination and respiration. When you breathe more deeply, you take in more oxygen and you get rid of more carbon dioxide and other waste products. In short, walking every day improves your general health and prolongs your prime of life.

When you walk, don't stroll. Go at a good brisk clip. But don't jog or run. Walk fast instead. How far you walk each day depends on you, how much spare time you have, that sort of thing. But once you start, keep it up. You'd be better off to walk half a mile each day than go five miles a day once a week.

If you don't like to walk, get a bicycle. Bicycling is a lot of fun, especially with a group. If you can't manage a two-wheeler, get a three-wheeler bicycle instead. That's the kind my wife uses and she really enjoys it.

To stay young, think young

If you want to stay young, think young. Associate with younger people if you want to keep from getting old. Stay away from those retirement communities where you have to be 55 or more to get in. Don't allow yourself to get involved with people who do nothing but sit around in rocking chairs and reminisce about yesterday. Yesterday is gone forever. Today, the ever-present now, is the only time that counts, no matter how old you are. A person who thinks young is enthusiastic about living. He is interested in learning something new every day no matter how old he is. He tackles life with the zest and curiosity of a child.

One of the youngest men I know is a friend of mine who is 76 years old. Mac is an accountant by profession. He worked for a large industrial firm until he was 65 and then he retired. After two years of loafing, sitting in a rocking chair and fishing, Mac gave up retirement as a bad job and went back to work.

He started a small bookkeeping service for small businessmen and kept their books on a weekly basis. Then he branched out into income tax service and decided to franchise his operation.

Today, his business is booming and his gross income is figured in six figures. But Mac is still up at six every morning and puts in a full work day. When people ask him why he continues to work as hard as ever, he replies, "I've never known hard work to kill anyone. More people rust out when they're old than wear out. Not me. I'll be damned if I'm going to sit around and rust out."

How You Can Gain These Benefits for Yourself

Calcium is one of the minerals most Americans lack in their diets, and iron is the other. You need at least 1,000 or 2,000 milligrams of calcium each day. When you're older, it may be necessary to go as high as 4,000 or 5,000 milligrams daily because calcium is often so poorly absorbed.

Calcium will keep your bones strong and prevent disabling fractures that happen so often to older people. It is also valuable for strong, firm and healthy fingernails. Don't worry about too much calcium causing kidney stones. Plenty of magnesium, which is found in dolomite, and pyridoxine (vitamin B-6) will keep that from happening. Your body must have plenty of calcium if you are to stay healthy.

* * *

Zinc is the vital element in maintaining a healthy prostate. If you're still young, start taking 30 milligrams of zinc each day while your prostate is still normal. Why wait until it's enlarged and painful before you do something about it? Zinc when you're young is the best way I know to avoid trouble with your prostate in later years, nor will it harm to take six bee pollen tablets a day, too. You might as well use every safeguard you can while you're still in good health.

* * *

In addition to Charlotte's methods of skin care, I would suggest these procedures to keep your skin from aging. Vitamin C will prevent many of the signs of older age: wrinkles, purple spots and skin hemorrhages. Too much sun over the years causes your face to become dry and wrinkled. Suntans may be fashionable when you're young, but they'll cause you all sorts of complexion problems when you're older. If you *don't* smoke, your face will have less wrinkles when you grow old. Women who smoke have more wrinkles in their forties that women who do not smoke have in their sixties.

* * *

Over the years, a great many herbs and exotic foods have been credited with improving sexual abilities. For instance, oysters have been said to help sexual performance, and rightly so. Why? Because they contain zinc. I have found zinc, vitamins E and F (the essential fatty acids) to be the three most influential foods in increasing sexual capacity. Do not buy your vegetable oils in the supermarket if you want to increase your sexual abilities. Buy only cold pressed oils that are sold in your health food store. The vegetable oils you see in the grocery store have been made by a chemical solvent process that leaves undesirable by-products in them.

* * *

Vitamin C is one of the vitamins that will prevent premature aging; vitamin E is the other. Lee's case is a good example of how vitamin E will help a person stay physiologically younger than his actual calendar years.

* * *

If you are in bad health and feel discouraged about your future just as Henry did, don't be. Get off the man-made carbohydrates of sugar and flour, eat natural foods as much as possible, and supplement your diet with natural vitamins and minerals. It will take time for your health to be restored. It won't happen overnight, but you will get better. I will discuss the vitamins and minerals my patients take after they are well in the next chapter so you'll know exactly what to take yourself.

What causes people to age prematurely and grow old before their time

People age faster than they should due to an excessive consumption of sugar. Sugar is a killer, and the sooner you eliminate it from your diet the better off you will be. Sugar upsets the metabolic processes in the body. That is a proven scientific fact. Excessive sugar intake continually stimulates the pancreas to produce insulin until it finally exhausts itself. You may not contract diabetes, but you will have an abnormal carbohydrate metabolism.

And when your carbohydrate metabolism is abnormal, you will age prematurely. You'll get old long before your time. Experiments at medical schools have shown that *people in their twenties who consume large amounts of sugar have the same kind of blood vessels as people in their seventies.* Their blood vessels have thicker walls and a narrower stream bed with resultant higher blood pressures.

No matter what your calendar age is, your physiological age will depend upon the condition of your circulatory system. Nowhere in the body is premature aging more evident than in the cardiovascular system.

If that information doesn't upset you, perhaps this will: male impotence is no longer a complaint limited only to gray-haired old men. It is now prevalent among young men due to the increased incidence of hypoglycemia. Doctors who have investigated abnormal carbohydrate metabolism have found that excessive sugar consumption causes male impotence at any age.

14

Outstanding Methods I Use
to Keep My Patients Well
After They Get Well

In the preceding chapters, I have emphasized several times that refined white sugar and bleached white flour, as well as all the packaged and processed foods containing them, are dangerous to your health. However, up to this point I have not offered you confirmation of that from other sources. I will do so right now.

Dr. Dennis Burkitt, of the Medical Research Council in London, England, has spent most of his professional career practicing medicine and doing research in South Africa. He says appendicitis, diverticulitis, cancer of the colon, gall bladder disease, hemorrhoids, obesity, varicose veins, blood clots in the veins and heart attacks are all results of a super-refined diet containing white sugar and white flour but lacking in fiber, cellulose, vitamins and minerals. As Dr. Burkitt points out, all these diseases are rare in rural Africa. They are, however, prevalent among urban Africans who changed their traditional primitive eating habits for those of "civilized" countries.

Dr. T. L. Cleave, also a famous and prominent British physician and scientist, has spent his life collecting evidence to prove that man-made carbohydrates, specifically refined white sugar and bleached white flour, are responsible for chronic and degenerative diseases. Dr. Neal Painter, Senior Surgeon at the Manor House Hospital in London, says that the refining of carbohydrates is a major cause of the ever-increasing death rate from heart disease.

Dr. John Yudkin, a distinguished British physician, biochemist, and researcher at London University says that sugar
plays a considerable part in all sorts of ailments including coronary heart disease, gastritis, hypoglycemia, obesity, complexion problems, tooth decay and eye conditions. In Canada,
Dr. Wilfrid Shute has been a pioneer in the use of vitamin E for
cardiovascular ailments. He is convinced that when modern
milling and baking methods removed the vitamin E from bread,
mankind was deprived of the one nutrient that could prevent
heart attacks and many other diseases of the circulatory system.

Here in the United States, Dr. E. Cheraskin, Professor and
Chairman of the Department of Oral Medicine at the University of Alabama, says the sugar-laden American diet has led to
a national epidemic of hypoglycemia and mental illness. He
says two technological "advances" have led to our super-refined
diet that is two-thirds man-made carbohydrates: one-third is
the milling process that gives us refined bleached white flour,
and the other is the processing of sugar cane into refined white
sugar. Dr. Cheraskin believes this kind of diet causes many of
our chronic degenerative diseases. Dr. W. M. Ringsdorf, Jr., is
an Assistant Professor of Oral Medicine at the University of
Alabama. He has co-authored many of Dr. Cheraskin's books
and shares his views on health and disease. Dr. David Reuben,
noted physician and author, blames refined white sugar and
ultra-refined white flour products for obesity and other chronic
diseases.

Foods my wife and I eat to stay healthy

When I was a boy growing up on a farm in the midwest,
supermarkets as we know them today did not exist. Most of
the vegetable produce sold in the corner grocery store —
potatoes, onions, carrots, lettuce, cabbage, tomatoes, corn,
beans — was grown by local farmers. We had our own garden
and ate good, fresh, healthful and wholesome food that was
filled with natural vitamins and minerals, unspoiled by preservatives, chemicals and excessive handling.

Today all that has changed. Almost every bite of food you
get now in the supermarket has been treated with chemicals

along the way — dyes, bleaches, emulsifiers, preservatives, antioxidants, flavor enhancers, buffers, acidifiers, alkalizers, naturalizers, gases, disinfectants, insecticides, defoliants, fungicides, artificial sweeteners, and heaven only knows what else. I am hard pressed to see how natural vitamins and minerals could survive that onslaught of chemicals.

Since I am not a chemist and I do not understand the meaning of all the terms I see on the labels of canned and packaged foods, I avoid the supermarket as much as possible and go to my local health food store instead. About all I buy in the supermarket are a few spices and condiments, eggs occasionally, and fresh meat. That's about the size of it. We no longer eat hot dogs, bacon, ham, or any other preserved meat since they contain *cancer-causing nitrates and nitrites.*

In the health food store I get my cereals — natural rolled oats, steel cut oatmeal, brown unpolished rice, cracked wheat, whole wheat, and unprocessed natural bran. These have no preservatives of any sort. I also buy stone-ground 100 percent whole wheat flour there. Since it, too, contains no additives or artificial chemicals to prevent spoilage, it must be kept in the refrigerator. I also buy stone-ground 100 percent whole wheat bread at the health food store. Sometimes, for variety's sake, I get a seven-grain loaf.

Since sugar is an absolute "no-no" at our house, *raw* honey takes its place. The honey you get at the supermarket has been cooked, pasteurized, and homogenized so it will not crystallize. Unfortunately, most of the natural nutrients were destroyed in the process. If my raw honey crystallizes, I place the container in a pan of water and *warm* it until the crystals go back into solution. I do not cook or overheat the honey.

The oil my wife uses for cooking, baking, and for salads is as *unrefined cold pressed* safflower or sunflower seed oil that contains no chemicals of any sort. The peanut butter we eat is ground from fresh peanuts right there before our eyes in the health food store. Again, no chemical preservatives or additives are used. The peanut butter you buy in the supermarket often contains *aflatoxin,* one of the most potent cancer-causing agents ever discovered.

Sea salt takes the place of ordinary table salt. It contains no calcium hydroxide to stabilize it, nor is there any calcium silicate to act as an anti-caking agent to make sure it always pours. Since cocoa and chocolate prevent the digestion and absorption of calcium from the digestive tract we use *carob*, a wholesome substitute for chocolate. It has none of the disadvantages of chocolate and cocoa, yet it has a rich taste that satisfies the sweet tooth we all have.

We are fortunate enough to live where roadside fruit and vegetable stands are found everywhere. We buy all our fresh produce from them, including farm fresh chickens, eggs and butter, in preference to the supermarket. I'm not saying their products are all free of harmful chemicals since frankly, I have no way of knowing. However, I do know that they haven't been further insulted with further unnecessary handling by wholesalers, retailers and other middle-men. That's about the best you can hope for in this age of ever-present chemicals. You can't avoid them all, but you can avoid as many of them as possible.

How to substitute natural foods for man-made artificial foods

You already know many of the substitutions I recommend for certain basic foods: whole grain cereals for boxed, sugary cereals; stone-ground 100 percent whole wheat bread and whole wheat flour for white bread and white flour; raw honey in place of refined white sugar; carob as a substitute for cocoa and chocolate.

However, that's only the beginning. I'm sure you have your own favorite recipes — perhaps handed down in the family for generations or passed on from friend to friend. Your familiar recipes can be made into the best natural food dishes simply by replacing those refined foods with the healthier and richer flavors of whole natural foods. It took a while to convince my wife to use honey instead of sugar and whole wheat pastry flour in place of bleached white cake flour in her baking, but now she wouldn't change back for anything. Here is a list of changes you can make to substitute natural foods for those disease-causing, man-made carbohydrates:

Leave Out	Substitute	Other Changes Required
All-purpose bleached white flour	Whole wheat flour or other whole grain flours	Requires more liquid
Bleached white cake flour	Whole wheat pastry flour	Requires more liquid
Baking powder	Low-sodium baking powder or active dry yeast	Use warm liquids
Chocolate and cocoa	Carob powder (equal amounts)	
Cornstarch	Whole wheat flour Brown rice flour Arrowroot powder	
Cracker or bread crumbs	Wheat germ or whole wheat bread crumbs	
Distilled vinegar	Apple cider vinegar	
Hydrogenated fats & shortenings	Unrefined oils, eg., sunflower or safflower	Requires more dry ingredients or less liquid
Refined oils	Unrefined oils	
Salt	Sea salt or kelp powder (equal amounts)	
Sugars	Raw honey (1 honey to 2 sugar)	Requires more dry ingredients or less liquid

To increase nutritional values, you can add noninstant dry milk powder, fresh wheat germ or nutritional yeast. Use liquid that is more nutritious than water whenever possible, such as fruit juice, vegetable stock or milk. Milk, yogurt and buttermilk are usually interchangeable; use yogurt instead of sour cream.

A few tips for cooking with natural foods

When you start using natural foods in your kitchen, I know you will want your meals to taste and look much as they always have. You can begin by substituting whole unrefined foods for refined ones and by eliminating white sugar and white flour from some of your favorite recipes. This can be done by using the substitution chart I've just given you.

You will soon find that your tastes are changing. As you begin to enjoy the many subtle flavors of whole foods, you will find it no longer necessary to sweeten and spice foods as heavily as before to give them flavor. Cooking will become a matter of combining natural flavors instead of seasoning foods to some preconceived taste. Simplicity is the key to developing a knowledge of cooking natural foods.

Here's a tip about how to cook natural cereals: the best way to cook steel cut oatmeal, for example, is to cover a cupful of oatmeal with hot water in a sauce pan. Let it soak overnight. In the morning, cook it only until the water is gone and the oatmeal is the consistency that you like. If you don't soak it all night, you would have to cook it for 30 to 45 minutes, and this would destroy some of the vitamin B complex and other food nutrients. You can use the same procedures for brown rice, cracked wheat or any whole grain cereal.

Pasta is another food well worth mentioning here, for many families are extremely dependent upon pasta in their meals. Macaroni, spaghetti and noodles made with whole grain flours are delicious and easy to cook. Once you taste them, you will never settle for anything less again. They also are available at your health food store.

Buckwheat Spaghetti is a blend of whole buckwheat flour

and soft wheat flour. Use it for a slightly different and refreshing flavor.

Whole Wheat Spaghetti and Macaroni are made of two varieties of wheat — unrefined durham wheat from North Dakota and Montana and soft wheat grown in the volcanic soils of eastern Washington. The whole grains are carefully ground into a fine textured flour made fresh for each batch of spaghetti. You can use this spaghetti in soups, casseroles and salads. Serve it with a meat and vegetable sauce, or fry it like Chinese noodles with vegetables.

Whole Wheat Flat Noodles are made of the same ingredients as whole wheat spaghetti. These noodles are excellent in vegetable casseroles. You can also make your own whole wheat noodles at home.

It is impossible for me to cover here all the information you need to cook with natural foods. I would suggest you get a good natural foods cookbook for a complete list of recipes. My wife uses Deaf Smith Country Cookbook, published by Macmillan Publishing Company, New York City. You can find it in any health food store.

How to keep from destroying vitamins and minerals in your kitchen

Vitamins and minerals can be lost in your kitchen by pouring the cooking water down the sink. B vitamins can also be destroyed by light and heat as well as baking soda and baking powder.

The key to the retention of these vitamins, minerals, enzymes and other food nutrients is to eat your fruits and vegetables raw whenever possible. If you cook your vegetables, don't overcook them. Prepare them Oriental style so they're still crisp and crunchy and can bite back at you. The less cooked your vegetables are, the more nutrition you'll get from them. The tops of many root vegetables, such as turnips, beets, carrots, and celery, contain valuable minerals, and should not be thrown away. They can be put through a juice extractor or blender, served as a cooked vegetable, or added to soup.

Raw foods are the secret to vigorous, long life

A good rule of thumb to follow is this: *if you can eat the food either raw or cooked, eat it raw.* I know it's necessary to have a hot vegetable such as potatoes, corn, beans, peas, and the like. I also know people cook vegetables that could be easily eaten raw and enjoyed. For instance, for years I never would have considered eating raw cauliflower. Then I tasted some with cheese dip at a party and I've eaten it raw ever since.

Raw fruits and vegetables are rich in vitamins, minerals and enzymes. They nourish the eyes and skin with vitamins A and C. Raw foods enrich the bloodstream with iron, copper, calcium and phosphorus. They are a powerful source of natural energy to your body.

Raw foods improve the appetite and do wonders for the digestive system. They put a rein on the urge for excessive seasoning. Raw fruits and vegetables provide bulk and cellulose, stimulate the muscular walls of the intestine, and provide healthful regularity without harmful laxatives.

How to buy foods in your supermarket and protect your health

1. *Avoid factory foods.* It may seem hard to you at first not to buy canned or packaged foods, but the more you replace them with fresh fruits and fresh vegetables, the better your health will be. Buy canned or packaged products only as a last resort.

2. *Never buy a food that will not spoil,* but eat it before it does. If you follow this simple rule, you'll never buy refined white sugar, bleached white flour, or any product made with them. Eat foods that are born — not foods that are made.

3. *Buy foods as often as possible.* Extra shelf life for canned and packaged goods is obtained by the use of chemical preservatives. That's a good reason not to buy them. *Your shelf life is important, too.* Don't overstock on your fresh fruits and vegetables. They will spoil before you can eat them. Besides,

storage causes a loss of vitamins, enzymes, and other valuable food nutrients.

4. *Eat foods that are in season.* Not only will they be less expensive for you to buy, but they will also have a richer supply of vitamins and minerals. This will also minimize the amount of preservatives used to keep the product fresh.

5. *Choose your supermarket carefully.* Cleanliness in handling fresh fruits and vegetables is a prime factor as far as I'm concerned. The closest big grocery store to me is less than a mile away, but I never go there because of its lack of proper sanitation. Instead, I drive nearly four miles to buy my food in a store that's kept spotless and scrupulously clean.

6. *Read the labels carefully.* Stay away from foods that have chemical sounding names on the label or that have such statements as "calcium propionate added to retard spoilage" — This is common in bread. BHA and BHT are chemical preservatives often used in boxed cereals.

7. *Avoid foods with "registered formulas" as much as possible.* The labels of packaged and canned foods are supposed to show a list of the ingredients they contain in *descending order* with the one having the most, first...the one having the least, last.

Unfortunately, this rule does not hold true for foods that have a *registered formula* with the government. These foods may list nothing at all or only some of the ingredients used. Foods that fall into this category include cocoa products... bleached white flour...macaroni, spaghetti, and noodles... white bread and rolls...enriched bread and rolls...raisin bread and rolls...milk and cream...processed cheeses... frozen desserts...food flavorings...salad dressings...canned fruit and fruit juices...canned vegetables...fruit pies...fruit butters...jams, jellies, and preserves...soft drinks.

The foolproof way to buy fruits and vegetables

Fruit

Buy fruit that is firm and fully ripened, but not overripe. Ideally, fruit should be left to ripen on the tree or the vine.

Unripened fruit should be kept at room temperature until it is soft.

The minerals in fruit are found just beneath the skin. They may be lost if the skin is removed. Sugar should never be added to fruit. If it is not naturally sweet enough, a little raw honey can be used.

The best way to be sure your fruit is of top eating quality is to buy when it's the cheapest. That means it's in season. Chances are it will be local produce which cuts down on shipping, storage and handling. If strawberries are going to be in season three months from now, wait a little, save some money, and get far better eating.

Apples can be digested raw by almost anyone. Your choice depends upon your taste: sweet, mellow or tart. Baldwin, Johnathan, Wealthy, Northern Spy, and York Imperial are excellent for every purpose. For eating or for salads, Delicious and Yellow Newtown are superb; Winesap, Rome Beauty, and Yellow Transparent are best for baking. A firm, unbroken skin is the key to quality. Good color appeals to the eye, but has no effect on the taste. Store apples at home in a cool place to keep them from spoiling.

An apple a day helps prevent tooth decay, says Doctor Harry E. Barnard, Chairman of the Food Division of the American Chemical Society. Dr. Barnard says an apple eaten in the evening will mechanically and chemically clean the teeth and protect them from bacterial ravages at night, when the most damage is done.

Bananas and pears should never be bought tree-ripened because they gain in natural carbohydrate content as well as becoming more tender after being picked. Bananas are at their best when they are a deep yellow flecked with tiny brown spots. Bananas that turn a brown color all over without flecking have been matured and ripened by gas. This makes them difficult to digest. Naturally ripened bananas are so easy to digest they can be given to babies as their first solid food. Pears need to be selected carefully. Hard pears will be gritty and bitter. Overripe pears will be soft and mushy.

Berries should be purchased without hulls except for

strawberries. You can judge the quality and taste by a firm, plump appearance and a rich color. *Grapes* and *cherries* can also be judged the same way. Large blueberries have a better flavor than smaller ones, but small strawberries usually taste sweeter than large ones. Check the box for evidence of staining, which is a sure sign the fruit is either overripe or moldy.

Grapefruit, an excellent source of vitamin C, is better judged by weight than by color or size. The average good grapefruit will be 75 percent liquid, so the weight is a good indication of the juice content. A grapefruit with smooth firm skin will have a much better flavor and more juice than a puffy coarse-skinned one.

Melons — big, juicy, and luscious — are considered to be the royalty of fruit. Although you can't look inside before you buy, you can tell a great deal about the quality from the outside by the look and feel of them so you won't be disappointed. And if you are a steady customer where you buy your fresh fruit and vegetables, you can always be sure of a free replacement when you get a bad melon.

Cantaloupe should have no trace of a stem at the blossom end when they are ripe. If the whitish netting covers the cantaloupe thickly and stands out with good definition like string or cord, then chances are good it will be a fine melon. A mature cantaloupe will have a sweet delicate aroma when it is ripe. If the outer skin is a deep yellow, it is probably overripe.

The bigger the honeydew, the better the taste. You can buy this melon even when it's hard, for it can ripen and mature in a warm moist area out of direct sunlight. The color should be creamy white or pale yellow, with a slight oily film on the outer surface.

Oranges and lemons should be thin skinned and heavy for the maximum amount of juice. Fruit that has been stamped *color added* should be avoided. The rind of the lemon can be good to use in scrubbing up and cleaning dirty elbows. It softens the skin and whitens the discoloration that comes from constant desk work.

Pineapples, when fully ripe, are golden colored and give off a sweet aroma. You can test the ripeness of a pineapple by pulling a spine away from its leafy top. When the pineapple is ripe, the spine will come away easily.

Vegetables

When buying vegetables, always select those that are well colored and free from signs of disease. Deficiency signs in vegetables are numerous and can be easily spotted, for instance, uneven ripening of tomatoes, wilted leaves on spinach, rust-colored streaks on lettuce, cracked centers of cabbage or cauliflower, and split stalks of celery. These blemishes can be found when the plant is deficient in minerals.

Use vegetables that are in season in preference to buying those that are canned or frozen. Just as with fruit in season, you'll be assured of better quality, and you'll save money too. Canning destroys most of the vitamins and enzymes. Although freezing vegetables is not as destructive to the vital food nutrients, each change of temperature still takes its toll.

Leafy Vegetables such as cabbage, cauliflower and lettuce are best when the head is heavy, compact, crisp and unspotted. The green outside leaves contain some of the most valuable nutrients.

Root Vegetables — carrots, beets, parsnips, radishes, turnips — should be young, firm, smooth and regularly shaped. The tops of turnips are extremely rich in vitamins and calcium. In Europe it is the custom for people to eat the turnip tops and for animals to eat the roots.

Onions in the store should feel dry enough to crackle. They should not have sprouts or split bulbs.

Peppers and Cucumbers should be firm, smooth, and have a deep attractive color. The peel of cucumbers is often sprayed or waxed, so it should not be eaten. The pepper is an excellent food, extremely high in vitamins.

Potatoes are an abundant source of vitamins and minerals. Buy those that are firm and free from cuts, growth cracks, deep eyes and knobby defects.

Well-shaped potatoes with shallow eyes keep waste to a minimum in preparation for cooking. "Sunburned" potatoes have a green surface color and usually taste bitter. Frost-damaged potatoes should be avoided, too. They usually have a watery, soggy appearance, or show a black ring near the surface when cut across.

Tomatoes should be fresh, firm, smooth and regularly shaped. If they are picked green they will soften with age, but they will not become juicier or tastier in the process. Tomatoes ripened artificially with gas are far inferior to those grown and ripened naturally out of doors. Canned or cooked tomatoes have much less food value than raw ones.

Vitamins and minerals I take and recommend for my own patients

I have no patience whatever with doctors who say you don't need to take vitamins and minerals if you eat a good balanced diet. Who eats a balanced diet every day of the week? Anyone? Very few people. Besides, how could you possibly expect to get a balanced diet when all the vitamins and minerals have been removed? Take "enriched" flour products, for instance. Over 20 *natural* nutrients have been removed, only four *artificial* ones put back in the manufacturing process. Not only that, such doctors base their ideas about vitamins on the information put out by the Federal Food and Drug Administration, whose tables show only the *minimum* daily allowance recommended for *healthy* people. That allowance is just about enough to keep a *sick* person breathing and that's all. I know that doctors who say vitamins and minerals won't cure disease have never used them in their practices. Had they done so, they would realize how valuable they are in restoring a person to health.

Most officials of the Food and Drug Administration, as well as those of the Food and Nutrition Board of the National Academy of Sciences, say their figures are only *"guesstimates,"* that they are based on animal experiments, and not on human experience. And since we are all different, no two of us can have the same exact vitamin demands, just as none of us has the same *minimal* requirements for water each day. Here's what I myself take each day and what I recommend for my own patients after they're well. As you can see, the figures are well above and beyond the minimum daily requirements of the

FDA. Incidentally, I myself always use the top figure of those listed.

Vitamin A	10,000-25,000 units
Vitamin D	400-1,200 units
Vitamin E	800-1,200 units
Vitamin C	1,500-5,000 milligrams

Vitamin B Complex: One to three capsules of a good vitamin B supplement such as B-100 will furnish the following each day:

Vitamin B-1 (Thiamine)	100-300 milligrams
Vitamin B-2 (Riboflavin)	60-180 milligrams
Vitamin B-3 (Niacin)	100-300 milligrams
Vitamin B-6 (Pyridoxine)	100-300 milligrams
Vitamin B-12	100-300 milligrams
Folic Acid	100-300 milligrams
Pantothenic Acid	100-300 milligrams
Biotin	100-300 milligrams
Para-Aminobenzoic Acid (PABA)	100-300 milligrams
Calcium	1,000-2,000 milligrams; 4,000 to 5,000 milligrams if elderly and poorly absorbed
Magnesium	In proportion with calcium in dolomite
Zinc	30 milligrams

Additional supplements I recommend to my patients besides those listed above are these: *dessicated liver tablets* and *brewer's yeast tablets.* They are potent sources of the B complex and fill any gaps that might be left. They are also a valuable source of protein. *Multimineral tablets* to supply iron, iodine, copper, potassium, manganese, and phosphorus...*sea kelp* to supply trace minerals...*lecithin* for nervous stability and fatty acid control — all these are taken as recommended by the individual manufacturer.

Why Norene is a healthy baby

Some of us may not be able to attain perfect health. We started too late and too much damage has been done. But those who start soon enough with natural foods, vitamins and minerals have a chance to be healthy all their lives. Take little Norene, for instance. She is the two-year-old daughter of two of my patients. They have decided to raise her solely on natural foods and not feed her any of the man-made carbohydrates.

Norene has never been sick a day in her life; she has not had so much as a runny nose. She has been brought up on plenty of fresh fruits and vegetables, wheat germ, yogurt, whole-grain bread and cereals and fresh milk. Her parents also add lecithin granules to her cereal. She receives the same vitamins and minerals her parents take (based on my recommended list), but in the proper amount for her size and age.

Norene has never tasted a piece of candy. Instead she munches on protein tablets or cookies made at home from stone-ground whole wheat pastry flour and raw honey. She has never had any refined white sugar or bleached white flour in her life.

Both parents feel the results are well worth the effort and I heartily agree. Norene may never have to suffer with the chronic and degenerative diseases you and I have had to put up with. By learning how to eat properly when she's young, she will form good eating habits that will stay with her for the rest of her life

Index